'Don't Sweat it *is not only packed with really good information but it's fun, interesting, and written from a personal point of view. Not at all preachy, it should be required reading for both women and men as soon as they reach forty. I feel like running down the street with this book screaming,* Viva la révolution!'

— Peta Mathias

'The menopause manual every Kiwi woman needs on the bedside table.'

— Kate Rodger

Nicky Pellegrino

Don't Sweat it

How to make 'the change' a good one

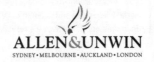

ALLEN&UNWIN
SYDNEY · MELBOURNE · AUCKLAND · LONDON

First published in 2022

Allen & Unwin
Level 2, 10 College Hill
Auckland 1011, New Zealand
Phone: (64 9) 377 3800

info@allenandunwin.com
www.allenandunwin.co.nz

83 Alexander Street
Crows Nest NSW 2065, Australia
Phone: (61 2) 8425 0100

A catalogue record for this book is available
from the National Library of New Zealand

ISBN 978 1 988547 81 7

Design by Saskia Nicol
Set in Freight
Printed and bound in Australia by Griffin Press

10 9 8 7 6 5 4 3 2 1

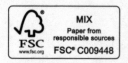

Contents

Chapter 1
Everyone was annoying

Everyone was *really, really* annoying. What was wrong with them all? And how was I supposed to cope? The tension of it, day after day, was making me clench my jaw so tightly it ached. A dentist told me I was grinding down my teeth. He said that all the clenching was overworking the muscles, too, so I was changing the shape of my jawline. My face looked squarer and more masculine, and my teeth were crumbling because every single person I had any dealings with at all was driving me crazy. That made me even *more* furious.

Then it occurred to me: I was the common denominator here. Other people had always been irritating; it was *me* who had changed. I had lost my ability to deal with it (which, to be fair, had never been especially well developed in the first place). I was in a towering rage most of the time, and distorting my own appearance as a consequence — not because of anything that was happening in the outside world, but due to the changes going on inside my own body.

Midlife and menopause: two words to strike fear in most women of a certain age. Words we'd rather not say out loud until we really have to. Because they mean we're getting older, and who wants to psychologically adjust to that?

We all know that at some point our ovaries will retire from active service and our hormones will go haywire. We've heard whispers of the side-effects, of hot flushes and mood swings, of dry vaginas and insomnia and night sweats. But like so much in life, menopause — and its stealthy harbinger peri-menopause — is something every woman experiences differently, so even if your mother, or an aunt, or an older female friend has attempted to initiate you, their descriptions of the biological realities of midlife might not match what you encounter.

My own mother's generation didn't really discuss it. They cryptically mouthed the words 'the change' at each other instead. And yes, it is a change. It's one that brings good as well as bad, one that might be tricky to deal with but can't, at this point anyway, be entirely avoided.

Nobody ever congratulates you for becoming meno-pausal, do they? But there is often so much excite-ment around every other life stage. Like the transition from girl to woman: your first bra, your first kiss, even your first experience of menstruation — it's new and wonderful, it feels like you're on the cusp of something great; people throw you parties, they give you special presents. And the deal is much the same when you start having babies: another welcome change, more cause for celebration.

Isn't midlife, in its own way, also a coming-of-age? Aren't you again on the cusp of something interesting? Unless things go very wrong, current life expectancies mean we're likely to be around for another 30 years or so after menopause/ruahinetanga. That is time for a lot of living. We may no longer be *re*productive, but we can still be productive. It's a milestone worth celebrating; at least, in my opinion.

Someone I was chatting to the other day mentioned being out with a girlfriend and heading into a bar when the friend happened to say that she was in the midst of a hot flush. 'I mean, really,' my (female) mate complained to me, wrinkling her nose in distaste. 'We were supposed to be out having a good time. I didn't want to hear about that.'

Well, in this book we're going to hear all about being hot, sweaty, angry, sad, itchy, anxious, bone-tired, fatter, vaguer, sleepless, wrinklier and drier of vagina. And I promise you we're still going to have a good time.

At no point will I tell you what to do — that's entirely up to you — but we will, with the help of experts, be taking a deep dive into the many options for managing the symptoms listed above. We'll investigate the stuff that no one ever tells you about midlife, celebrate as well as commiserate, and we'll meet other women, get their perspective and talk this thing through.

~

Life can be even better once the hormonal storm subsides. Women who no longer shop for tampons are out there running countries and businesses, acting in hit Hollywood movies, writing award-winning books, crashing through glass ceilings. It isn't always easy, but then what is? By the time we hit midlife we've weathered a lot of other storms — so we've got this, really we do.

There may be a few freaky moments along the way. When I was at the dizzying heights of rage and my brain seemed not to fully belong to me anymore, a man in a grocery store made the mistake of accusing me of queue-jumping. In my defence, there was a confusing set-up in this particular shop and he was possessed of (irritatingly!) poor queuing skills. I hadn't meant to jump ahead. But as I began to apologise, he declared that he thought I was very rude and so did everyone else. 'I'll show you rude,' I thought to myself. And then I did.

Afterwards, once I'd recovered from being a lot stroppier than the situation demanded, I considered designing a range of humorous menopause slogan T-shirts to make women with swinging moods easier to identify. Then I googled, and there are already loads out there. Unfortunately most are a bit lame, although I did like the one that said 'I'm hot, I'm cold, I'm hot, I'm cold, IT'S YOUR FAULT!'

So yes, I'm menopausal. I've been there, done that, although I don't yet have the T-shirt (and if I did it would need to be in a larger size with longer sleeves).

~

Midlife changes us in ways we never imagine. Sometimes it feels as if we're rebuilding ourselves from the ground up. This new version of us — what will we want, and who are we going to be? I guess it's time to find out.

'I've decided there can't be many menopausal women in hell because they wouldn't put up with it. They'd band together, overthrow the Devil and get the air-conditioning turned up.'

— Karen Mills, comedian

Chapter 2

And then the menopause stole my wardrobe

I have just stripped off my dress, kicked off my sneakers and am sitting at my desk in nothing but a tiny slip. Thankfully I work at home, not in an office, but the occupants of six other neighbouring houses could potentially be getting an eyeful. Never have I cared less about anything.

The hotness of a hot flush is not like any other sort of warmth. It comes from deep within. Often for me it starts with a spike of anxiety (more on that later), then the heat rushes over me in a wave and I feel stifled by it. There's always a moment when my skin feels as if it has been packed in warm clay, but thankfully I don't get sweaty so if it weren't for the sudden manic stripping-off of clothes then probably no one would guess what was happening.

Ah yes, clothes. The change of midlife has even extended to them. I'm trying to clear out the things that don't suit me anymore and it's taking a toll on my psyche. Since I'm not a huge shopper, a lot of those outfits have been mine for a long time. Each garment that goes into the bag to be taken to an op shop carries memories of the younger woman who used to wear it, the one who felt good in sleeveless, backless, even body-hugging fashion. It's a slow process, this saying goodbye to the clothes that the menopause has stolen from me. Sometimes I snatch things back from the departure area and restore them to their original spot in my wardrobe. I like those clothes. I had good times in them. It seems unreasonable that they don't like me anymore.

It's not that I've gained a huge amount of weight; it's more like all the fat in my body got together for a party and afterwards couldn't find the way back to its proper home. So instead, it settled in other spots — my stomach, my back — and just sort of thickened me in places that were never thick before.

I can still fit into most of the things I'm getting rid of. There's no law against exposing your upper arms after the age of 50, so I could try to love the cellulite-like effect that's visible on them in brighter lights. Eventually my whole body is going to be pleated like an Issey Miyake dress, so I may as well get used to it. But right now I only want to wear things that I look my best self in. They need to flow past my body rather than cling to it, and cover as much of my arms and legs (veins, cellulite, weird lumpy bits, etc.) as possible. And so I'm saying goodbye to a lot of strappy tops and my favourite black crêpe wrap dress. Deep down inside I still feel like the woman who wore them, the one whose slim arms and great shoulders were her best features, but the mirror is telling me a very different story.

~

I'm trying to enjoy the process of redefining my style, but it's fair to say that there have been a few false starts. At one point I decided it would be a good idea to free myself from the tyranny of grooming, so had my longish hair cut into a sensible bob. Then, on a night out with a group of same-life-stage friends I realised that literally every single one of us had the same haircut. This seemed faintly sinister. Like we were turning into middle-aged clones.

My initial attempts to streamline a new utilitarian midlife wardrobe also misfired. I decided that I was going to exist in a pared-down uniform of almost identical clothes — a tactic employed by the likes of Barack

Obama and Steve Jobs to free their minds to focus on more important things, which surely contributed to their success. 'Yes, but they were both already geniuses,' a helpful friend pointed out. 'Looking really boring isn't going to turn you into one.'

And she had a point. Why would I choose for my personal style to be dull just because alien flesh has attached itself to my middle and I'll never again wear a top tucked into a waistband? Why shouldn't I look nice? Indeed glamorous, if I'm in the mood for it? Maybe even sexy?

Older women actually are allowed to be sexy, but only if they play by the rules. French women are skilled at this. Vanessa Paradis, Isabelle Huppert, Juliette Binoche, Audrey Tautou, Charlotte Rampling (English, but has lived in Paris for decades). Google Carine Roitfeld, the former editor of French *Vogue*. She wears a look that is apparently acceptable at any age — pencil skirt, silk shirt, biker jacket — because it is chic sexy.

No one criticises Michelle Obama for being timelessly elegant. Or Dame Kiri Te Kanawa for mastering the art of smart-casual classic. But overstep the line, edge towards overtly sexy, and the judgements will come and they will be gleeful.

Just look at the pasting Madonna got when she showed up on a TV chat show (*The Graham Norton Show*) wearing a bustier. Yes, there was a lot of pillowy breast on show and she had accessorised with an eye patch, which seemed eccentric. Online forums lit up with misogyny and ageism: she was ridiculous, a total idiot, ugly, tragic. Actually, she was in costume. Plus, this is a woman who has spent every decade of her life so far being creative and pushing the boundaries. If she wants to whip out her cleavage and show a lot of leg, shouldn't that be up to her? Does Madonna really deserve to be cancelled for looking sexy in her sixties?

There are a few preternaturally youthful women like J.Lo and Halle Berry who seem to get away with baring midriffs and cleavage, but they are the exceptions. Remember how New Zealand TV presenter Hilary Barry was scolded for baring one shoulder? 'Please encourage Hilary to dress properly,' complained a viewer. 'Exposed shoulders are for the young.'

My cleavage long ago retired from public life, and I'm okay with that. But I reserve the right to be sexy in my late fifties and for as long as I damn well feel like it. Why should foxiness be the province of the young? Whose decision was *that*?

Unfortunately, fashion designers aren't doing everything they can to help the midlife woman. A lot of them might prefer it if we didn't use their clothes to skim rounded bellies, conceal swollen knees, cover dimpled arms and veil wrinkled cleavage. Once, for a magazine article, I interviewed a designer (of expensive, high-quality clothes) who begged me not to give her age because she didn't want to turn younger customers off. That designer might have been missing a trick. A great many middle-aged women have more spending power than ever before in their lives. If we care about looking good, we can afford to.

~

While age is changing the way we look, inside we still feel young. It's only when I catch sight of myself unexpectedly in a mirror and wonder what my mother is doing there, that I'm reminded of what time is doing. I was never beautiful — as in so many other areas of my life, I was always just kind of average. But I did notice the moment when I became quite invisible. It wasn't that I missed being wolf-whistled at when I walked past building sites — more that suddenly I realised that people were looking past me, blocking my way or even crashing into me. I'm 1.85 metres tall, a skyscraper of a woman and easily spotted, but suddenly I was like some sort of zombie life-form walking unseen among the masses.

It really hit home one night when I visited a downtown Auckland bar, one of those places that is full of wealthy guys, glamorous women and gorgeous young bar staff. Neither me nor my fortysomething friend could get served. We might have died of thirst except that I waylaid a barman, saying 'Excuse me, but who do I have to fuck to get a drink round here?' I have never seen a person pour two glasses of wine faster. He was wide-eyed and visibly pale. Possibly he is now getting therapy.

It seems to me that a woman today has two, maybe three, routes to take. She can enter midlife looking like she actually belongs there, so a bit frayed around the edges and effectively invisible. Or she can fight for visibility with every weapon at her disposal, restricting calories, doing all the exercise, smoothing wrinkles and plumping lips with Botox and filler, and then risk being labelled a cougar and vain. The third possible option is to go down the *Advanced Style* route. This is the name of a blog by New Yorker Ari Seth Cohen that showcases older people who are stylish and often flamboyant, like the very fabulous Iris Apfel. I did try route three for a time. I bought lots of bright bangles, a bold necklace and a pair of purple suede boots, but I couldn't pull it off. In the words of Lady Gaga, you have to be born this way.

~

The modern menopausal woman has it easier than her nineteenth-century Pākehā counterparts who, with their changing bodies, and hairier chins and upper lips, were considered to be unwomanly viragos. Menopause back then was viewed, at least in some cultures, as the decline of life, a time to be dreaded, and becoming unattractive to men was an unprecedented disaster in any female's life.

Don't Sweat it

The male gaze isn't quite so celebrated these days. We're not supposed to want it as much. The modern feminist view is that the way a man views a woman shouldn't define her, and I think we're all behind that 100%. But lots of midlife women I've spoken to said they had enjoyed their time basking in the male gaze and they missed it now. One woman described walking down a street and realising that not a single passing man had bothered to glance her way. 'They stepped around me as if I were a lamppost. It was like a slap in the face,' she told me.

Others admitted to worrying that they were losing their value along with their youthful beauty. 'If a woman is a trophy, then what happens once she is tarnished?' asked one. Did you gasp, reading that? I'll admit I had a sharp intake of breath when she said it. I can't say that I've ever thought of myself as a trophy. But I have spent decades wishing that I was thinner and prettier, with glowier, unblemished skin and no cellulite. Blame the patriarchy, my upbringing, the beauty industry or glossy magazines, it doesn't much matter — I didn't stop wishing for any of those things just because I turned 50.

Many midlife women I spoke to missed looking good effortlessly. Being attractive was a part of who they were, and now it took a lot more time and work before they could smile at themselves in a mirror. Not everyone feels like this, obviously, and I did speak to women who weren't remotely worried what they looked like — but they were the rarer ones.

While appearance might not be the *most* important thing, it still is important. And invisibility tends to come along at the same time as a series of other events. Fertility declines, kids leave home, parents age and die. All of which coincide with a change in oestrogen and progesterone levels bringing on the symptoms of peri-menopause. You gain weight, you sweat, you burn, you palpitate; your *body odour* changes, for goodness' sake. You get anxious, you lose your confidence, you can't sleep, your fingernails break and your muscles ache. The least you could ask for is a good hair day, but it's greying and thinning, so good luck with that. (Here's a life hack you won't find anywhere else. If you're one of those people who always deletes the unflattering photos of them-selves, then don't. Keep a few for a more realistic future reference, so that when you're looking back you don't think 'OMG I was a supermodel then, what's happened to me?')

~

It's very easy to blame everything on hormones at this time of life. *I'm bloated* . . . bloody menopause . . . *I'm angry* . . . bloody menopause . . . *I'm tired* . . . bloody menopause . . . *I have a headache* . . . bloody menopause . . . *I keep sneezing* . . . bloody menopause. There can be other reasons for all those things and it's worth exploring them, but chances are that whatever the source of the problem, hormonal chaos will be making it worse.

Don't Sweat it

The menopause transition sneaks up on you. Perhaps your periods get heavier and more irregular, or your skin gets a bit itchy, or some days you feel tearful for no reason. Probably this starts to happen in your forties, but potentially it begins earlier and it's very easy to miss what's going on. It's not as if a piece of ticker-tape comes out your ear saying 'You're officially peri-menopausal, expect shit to happen.' Perhaps you always had bad PMT, or endometriosis or terrible menstrual flooding. Maybe your skin was always sensitive and your moods a bit swingy. If you're really busy, then naturally you'll feel exhausted. If you're stressed, you can't sleep. If your partner is driving you crazy, then obviously you won't want to have sex with him. And that's how the change can begin without you really noticing.

I can't pinpoint when my peri-menopause began exactly, but looking back there were signs that I missed at the time. I started to get a sensation like the skin all over my body was itching and crawling. One day I was at a friend's place and I could hear her kids playing but couldn't see them — that entire spot in my vision was missing. I thought I'd had a stroke, so it came as a relief when my head started to hurt and I realised it must be a migraine. Oh yes, and the other thing — please look away now if you're squeamish — the spectacular menstrual clotting. One clot was so big I thought I'd lost a minor organ.

Because I was busy, I tried not to think about any of it too much. As a journalist I reported on health for years while wilfully ignoring my own. This affected my life — my periods were brutal, my iron levels plummeted, I got sick more easily as a result, and there was at least one day a month when I had to remain within 100 metres of a toilet.

I used to feel solidarity with other women I came across in workplace lavatories who were tearfully trying to scrub the leakages of blood from the backs of skirts and trousers. 'I've been there,' I'd say, offering them free access to my desk-drawer stock of giant-sized pads and super tampons. We were a secret society, us heavy bleeders, although hopefully that is changing. The actor-turned-lifestyle-guru Gwyneth Paltrow spoke in a Goop podcast about her peri-menopausal flow being so heavy she once had to wear a sweater tied around her waist to get off a plane.

If I had a time machine, then on the way back to assassinate Hitler and persuade Donald Trump's mother to use birth control I would stop off and whisk my younger self to the gynaecologist who had suggested I have a Mirena inserted. This hormonal intra-uterine device releases small amounts of levonorgestrel, a synthetic progestogen, which reduces the monthly growth of the lining of the womb and so reduces the monthly blood loss (it's also an effective contraceptive). Despite having friends who said it changed their lives, I hesitated because it seemed icky. Now I would grab the chance to give my past self a decent talking to and explain a few of the things I've learned over the intervening years about what goes on inside a peri-menopausal woman's body.

'Peri-menopause and menopause should be treated like the rites of passage that they are. If not celebrated then at least accepted and acknowledged and honoured.'

— *Gillian Anderson,* People *magazine*

Chapter 3

It's all about oestrogen (and hotness)

Oestrogen is like one of those quiet, conscientious workers who achieve a lot without any fuss, and only when they walk out of the job do you realise how much they did. This hormone is a multi-tasker: there are oestrogen receptors on cells all over the body — in the brain, your skin, your vagina and vulva, your bladder wall, etc. Not only is oestrogen helping to regulate your menstrual cycle, but it's also helping to keep your skin firm and your brain supplied with the feel-good chemical serotonin. It affects your bones, heart and blood vessels, mucous membranes, hair and breasts, and reproductive tract. When you've got the right amount of oestrogen, steadily and surely doing its thing, then you barely notice.

However as the ovaries begin to wind down, this affects production of the hormone. The problem is that oestrogen doesn't just slide into a graceful swan dive, it roller-coasters up and down. Sometimes you have too little and sometimes too much. Although I didn't realise it at the time, the migraines I began to have out of the blue were a sign that my oestrogen was fluctuating. I did feel slightly better after talking to Christchurch endocrinologist Anna Fenton, who admitted that she got migraines once or twice a month for a couple of years before working out what was going on. Hormones are her job, but she still managed to miss it. 'Sometimes I'd vomit into a basin between patients and then carry on,' she said. 'Then finally the penny dropped.'

~

There are three types of oestrogen in the female body. *Oestriol* is produced by the placenta and rises in pregnancy to help the uterus grow and prepare for birth. *Oestradiol* is mainly produced by the ovaries and is the really good stuff that your body loves and has to learn to do without in midlife. In post-menopausal women, the oestrogen found in higher quantities is called *oestrone*. It's produced in the fatty tissue and the adrenal glands as well as the flagging ovaries, but it's weaker and won't make up for the loss of all that oestradiol.

Oestrogen rises and falls in a fairly predictable way during all your years of menstrual cycling, but in midlife it goes haywire and there's no real way to keep track of it. At one time there was a trend for peri-menopausal women to have a series of blood tests in a bid to keep tabs on hormone levels. However, in peri-menopause your oestrogen levels can surge and decline within just 24 hours, so a blood test is only going to give you a snapshot of what the oestrogen is like at that particular moment in time.

Two other relevant hormones, follicle-stimulating hormone (FSH) and luteinising hormone (LH) are made by the pituitary gland and involved in ovulation, and both are elevated during peri-menopause and menopause. The experts I spoke to said that testing is useful if someone is young to be having symptoms or when other causes for those symptoms are suspected. But for most midlife women with obvious symptoms, these tests are probably surplus to requirements.

No expert I consulted was a fan of salivary hormone testing. The Australasian Menopause Society says there is no evidence that results will be accurate or useful, and doesn't endorse the use of these tests. Some practitioners of alternative medicine use the DUTCH test (it stands for dried urine test for comprehensive hormones), which is a strip you dip in your pee that will measure things like cortisol, testosterone and melatonin levels as well as oestrogen. The DUTCH test isn't standardised in the same way as laboratory blood tests. Also it costs several hundred dollars, whereas blood tests are free in Aotearoa New Zealand.

If what you're interested in is your fertility — what your egg reserves are looking like and when menopause seems likely to arrive — then the test you want is the one for anti-Müllerian hormone (AMH), which is secreted by the ovarian follicles. In most parts of the country this blood test is not funded as a predictor of menopause, but it is relatively inexpensive and commonly used by fertility specialists to help them assess where a woman is at.

By the time your periods are all over the place and you're so sweaty at night that you sleep on a towel and you're even yelling at the cat, you don't need any tests to tell you that you're in the menopause transition. If you're anything like me, then you might soldier on ignoring all the other peri-menopausal signs for quite some time. But if and when the hot flushes strike, even the most oblivious or in-denial woman is going to realise what is going on.

~

It's worth examining the anatomy of a hot flush. First of all, we don't completely understand what's going on with them — a surprisingly common occurrence with women's health in general and menopause in particular. With flushes, what we do know is that it has to do with oestrogen's action on the brain, specifically the hypothalamus. This is a small region at the base of the brain that plays a crucial role in many functions, including regulating your temperature.

Usually our bodies have a very efficient thermoregulation system. If the temperature around you drops, you don't shiver until it becomes very cold; and if it rises, you don't sweat until it becomes very hot. In menopause, that window shrinks. The hypothalamus, somehow confused by the drop in oestrogen, triggers an unnecessary heat reaction. Your heart pumps faster, the blood vessels in your skin dilate to circulate more blood and radiate off the heat, and your sweat glands release moisture to cool you further.

You may not get any hot flushes at all, and if you do they might be major or minor. And heat isn't necessarily the whole story. Here's a thing I didn't know until it happened to me — hot flushes are typically accompanied by a surge of adrenaline, and so there can be a few moments before a flush where things get weird. It might feel like a sudden spike of anxiety; you might get a racing heart or quite severe palpitations. At one stage my pre-flush palpitations were so bad that I blacked out and almost fainted. The first time I was at my desk, but the second time I was walking through a park and had to push past several people, fling myself down on a bench and shove my head between my knees.

I was 90% sure the cause was my hot flushes — but the other 10% of me was worried that there was something very wrong with my heart, and it was this 10% that kept waking me up in the middle of the night and freaking me out. So I took myself off to a cardiologist just to be on the safe side. He was a man of very mature years and must have seen rather a lot of middle-aged female patients in his career. When I told him about the palpitations and said I thought it might be a menopause symptom, he looked at me as if I was deranged. 'Don't you get other women my age complaining of the same thing?' I asked. He fixed me with that same look again and just said 'No.'

And so I wore one of those heart monitor things for 24 hours, and sure enough my heart was racing and, no, there was nothing wrong with it, and the cardiologist sent me away. My GP — a woman — agreed that this was most likely a precursor to a hot flush and prescribed beta-blockers, which I took for a few days and then stopped because actually just knowing that it was nothing serious had helped enough. Also, I read that beta-blockers can cause weight gain and I'm quite capable of that without any extra help.

So if you get the palpitations, by all means get checked — but maybe choose your cardiologist more carefully than I did. And if you get the weird anxiety thing, I feel your pain.

~

As for the actual hot flush, from my entirely unscientific research (talking to a lot of middle-aged women about it)

I can tell you that these vary widely. How often you get them, how long they last, whether you sweat, tear off your clothes — there are no rules.

For myself, I don't think there are any external signs that I'm having one although it's very obvious on the inside. There are women who go bright red in the face. Some women literally have perspiration flying off them, while others radiate a lot of heat but stay dry. 'At least they'll keep you warm in winter,' I've heard people say. But actually that's not how it works, because after you get hot you then get cold, and at night if you've sweated into your sheets or PJs you'll wake up soaked and shivery. There are no up-sides to continual outbreaks of feeling like a furnace, so let's stop pretending.

As with so many aspects of midlife, at least we have the comfort of solidarity. One woman described being at a dinner with a large group of same-age female friends. 'At any point in the evening someone was putting a cardigan on and someone was taking one off. Someone was opening a window and someone was closing one,' she said.

Up to 80% of women get flushes, flashes or whatever you want to call them. Some women feel dizzy or nauseous, some get a headache, some feel like the blood is rushing around their body — and this can potentially happen several times an hour. There is no knowing in advance how intense hot flushes are going to be for you. Last century some physicians believed that temperament played a part. They thought that a gentle, feminine woman would have a milder menopause than a virile, bold and energetic one — basically the message there was 'Be good and you won't suffer so much'. Amazingly, we haven't really progressed much further than that.

There is one theory that you're likely to have a similar menopause experience to the one your mother had, but I'm not sure how well that stands up. My mother claims not to have noticed hers happening and I definitely am noticing mine, so I suspect it's not that simple.

The list of potential triggers for the vasomotor symptoms (fancy term for flushes and night sweats) of menopause include quite a lot of things I consider necessities. Like coffee, wine and spicy food, which are well known as hot-flush enablers. Hot baths, hot drinks, blow-drying your hair and doing cardiovascular exercise can also set one off. Smoking makes flushes worse (there are officially NO health benefits to smoking, and I'm very grateful I never started), as does being overweight. I definitely notice that if I get very stressed suddenly, then it brings on a flush.

Very often there is no obvious reason at all. The flushes just happen, and keep happening for an average duration of 7.4 years after menopause. It is thought that women who start flushing before their final menstrual period may have the most persistent symptoms. Some have symptoms lasting for twelve years or more. Skinny, nondrinking, un-caffeinated women who never eat a curry can keep on flushing well into their seventies and beyond — so if you want that flat white or lamb vindaloo then you may as well have it.

~

The other issue with plummeting/spiking oestrogen is that you can be fooled into thinking that you've had your last period, throw a party, drink champagne (kidding, obviously) — and then a couple of months later, there it is again. I had some long gaps during which I rashly considered chucking out all my tampons, but next minute back it came, often in spectacular 'someone build an ark' fashion. Even double-bagging at night — wearing the largest available tampon and a thick pad — was not enough to stem the tide.

I will never forget my final period. It happened during the first national Covid-19 lockdown, and inconveniently I had broken my ankle so was unable to drive to the supermarket. For the first time in our almost 30 years together, my husband had to go shopping for my sanitary protection. We did a session on Google looking at pictures of my preferred brands, and then I sent him off with the instruction to buy what he considered to be a ridiculous amount and then buy even more. I needed them all.

And then, finally, it was over: 44 years of menstruation,

a whole lot of bleeding. Having been child-free by choice, I didn't mourn the end of my fertility and couldn't have been happier to see the last of my periods. But some women I spoke to experienced it as a huge loss. They grieved for their menstrual cycle and felt an altered sense of self without it. For some it cut deep because they'd never had all the children they longed for. For others, being fecund was tied in with being desirable and having power as a woman. Being able to save all the money they'd once invested in tampons and fearlessly wear white trousers was no consolation at all.

Maybe that seems like an over-reaction, because it's inevitable, right? It's going to happen to all of us, so there's no point getting upset about it. As a younger woman, you might think that you'll navigate the end of your fertility without too much trouble, but at that stage you've got oestrogen oozing all over those receptors in your brain. During the menopause transition, as oestrogen see-saws and then finally dips for good, your brain may struggle to adjust. At that point you're not going to take kindly to anyone who makes the mistake of saying you're over-reacting. There may not be blood, but there will be rage.

Chapter 4

And then the menopause stole my personality (or at least borrowed it)

It felt like I had imposter syndrome, except that the person I was pretending to be was myself — the me I *used* to be: the one who was mildly irritated at times, not constantly boiling over with rage. The me who didn't cry without cause or get anxious for no reason, or feel paralysed by inertia one minute and ready for anything the next.

Often I wondered whether people could tell from the outside that I'd gone loopy, because it was certainly obvious on the inside. Then I realised I wasn't alone; far from it. Others looked no different than before, and they sounded the same, but once I started asking questions almost every midlife woman I spoke to felt that their personality had changed in some way.

'I've lost my confidence' — that was what I heard most often. Beautiful, successful middle-aged women said it to me. Women I had known for years, and considered over-confident if anything. Women who had huge careers and on paper ought to have been peaking. They had left jobs because they couldn't cope anymore. Turned down opportunities. Or they were struggling to do what they'd easily managed before. They seemed bewildered, these women. Some of them were angry. This doesn't happen to men, one pointed out — a man's confidence seems only to increase as he follows the arc of his working life.

While I was researching midlife confidence loss, I happened to be on a radio panel show and among the topics of the day was an item on companies needing more females on their boards. I asked the expert if there was a shortage of women for these positions because some of them fall by the career wayside due to motherhood or 'they get menopausal and can't cope'. There was a furious reaction from listeners who thought I was being insulting and offensive.

To be clear, I'm not saying that all menopausal women will suffer flagging self-confidence. Many will forge ahead in their careers through any symptoms they happen to have. Helen Clark, pointed out one listener (yes, thanks, I *had* heard of her). But another sent a message saying that not too long ago she might have found what I said offensive 'but now I understand completely'.

~

Increasingly it's being accepted that in midlife some women go through a period of struggling or second-guessing themselves. For many this hits at the peak of their careers, and instead of recognising that hormones are the issue, they assume that they are stressed, over-busy or losing their minds.

In Australia, a survey by an employee benefits platform called Circle In found that almost half of women struggled with loss of confidence and worried about having to hide the fact that they were menopausal. A massive 83% felt that it had negatively affected their work and 70% weren't comfortable talking to their manager about it. That was a survey of 714 people, and I suspect it is pretty representative.[1]

I worked in female-dominated offices for years. My colleagues talked about their pregnancies, their PMS and even their period pains . . . but never did I ever hear anybody mention that they were menopausal.

In another survey by My Menopause Doctor, nine out of ten women said that their menopausal or peri-menopausal symptoms had a negative impact on their work — 9% had gone through a disciplinary process as a result of poor performance, 51% had reduced their working hours and 32% considered quitting their job altogether.[2]

Thoroughly modern workplaces are starting to be more supportive, or at least trying to break the taboo. A few are taking practical measures, such as having fans available or relaxing the rules around uniforms for women affected by hot flushes. Others are changing the culture at a deeper level, with more flexible working and better communication. But — so far — not many.

In a survey that Aotearoa's Gender Justice Collective released in 2020,[3] fewer than 1% of the respondents said that their workplace had a specific policy around menopause, 67% didn't, and 31% of respondents didn't know whether there was one or not — but 72% of the people who did the survey thought it was important that there be menopause policies in workplaces.

In New Zealand a woman called Jeanette Kehoe-Perkinson has set up an organisation called Power Pause. She goes into workplaces and talks all things menopause, helping women and their colleagues navigate the transition so that talented and experienced workers don't leave jobs because they are temporarily not coping quite as well. Jeanette's personal experience inspired Power Pause, and this is her story.

~

Jeanette Kehoe-Perkinson

'Part of me felt like a victim, and it's never good to feel like that.'

Jeanette is one of those warm, sunny, self-assured people who can make friends and connections very easily, and I'm pretty sure her personality is what fuelled her success in corporate human resources and executive development. She was in her forties when she started having night sweats and friends told her 'Welcome to peri-menopause.' Living in the UK at the time, working in a high-level job, she went on a combined (oestrogen and progesterone) hormone replacement (HRT) pill called Elleste Duet.

But then Jeanette moved to New Zealand with her family, where eventually she took a senior job at a bank. Elleste Duet isn't available in this country, so when her supply ran out, Jeanette ought to have gone to her doctor and asked for the best alternative, but she didn't.

'I was too busy — I didn't make time for myself and my health, and I take full accountability for the professional consequences,' she says.

Not only did she start having hot flushes in the boardroom, but there was also a seismic shift mentally.

'I couldn't remember words . . . I had brain fog and started getting anxiety,' she recalls. 'I've never had anxiety, ever. I was super-confident about my own ability, then suddenly it wasn't there anymore. Things I used to be able to do relatively easily I was really struggling with, and I was having to work harder, putting in ridiculous hours to keep up, and having fairly frequent mood swings.'

Her colleagues hadn't known Jeanette for very long, so had no idea that those mood swings weren't typical; that in fact they were really weird for her. Meanwhile she was reeling, because she could never tell what might trigger a surge of impatience, and she didn't understand that her hormone levels were the real cause.

'It just wasn't me,' she says. 'I'm a really happy person, and I care about other people and always want to do the right thing, so the mood swings were really confusing and probably damaged me the most because they affected some of my most important working relationships.'

Finally Jeanette left her job. The next day she went to see her doctor, in tears because she thought she had early-onset dementia. Fortunately the GP saw what Jeanette had managed to miss, and prescribed oestrogen patches and progesterone tablets to control her menopause symptoms.

'The HRT was a total game-changer,' she says. 'Within a week I got my energy back, felt like myself again and have been feeling terrific ever since.'

Jeanette's life had been radically changed, however, because she had stepped down from an executive job that was well within her usual capabilities.

'I've spent hundreds of thousands of dollars throughout my career investing in women's development programmes,' she says. 'I've tried to promote women through to leadership roles and to elevate their professional profiles. And then for me to suddenly fall, and know that there are influential people out there who think I'm a basket case or somehow moody, when I'm really not. I thought, Holy smoke, I can't let that happen to other people.'

And so Power Pause was born, as a social

enterprise that Jeanette fits around her other work as a chief people officer, along with board roles and executive coaching. It takes her into businesses where she gives a presentation to male and female employees, talking about her own experience and sharing the information they need about menopause. The idea is that a culture of openness will help keep women's careers on track. But also, as she points out, men who attend those presentations may have wives/partners, relatives and friends going through the menopause transition, so this is knowledge that can help prevent damaged relationships at home as well as in the workplace. Most importantly, it raises awareness and gives practical tips on how to support team members, retain talented women and show empathy in the workplace.

'I think the biggest thing that I'm trying to say is "this passes". If you're not supported it can be horrendous, and many people do get to a really dark place. In nations which track such statistics, such as the US, UK and Australia, women in their late forties to early fifties have the highest suicide rate after the teenage years. But like puberty, menopause is a life stage that you get through and then your memory comes back and your energy comes back. Once you've been through menopause it's a second spring — the next phase of your life — and it's brilliant.'

And then menopause stole my personality (or at least borrowed it)

There has been only positive feedback from the organisations Jeanette has worked with, via webinars or in-person workshops. One Australian company was worried about the implications of raising the subject of menopause in case people felt targeted and uncomfortable, but Power Pause is about increasing awareness for *all* genders and age groups, not just the women who are going through it. And while some people have thought that she was crazy to put herself out there, Jeanette has no regrets about going public with her own hormonal storm.

'That experience was so bad,' she says. 'Part of me felt like a victim, as I had zero workplace support, and it's never good to feel like that. But if it hadn't been as traumatic as it was, I never would have started Power Pause, never would have carved out the much-improved life I have now, and never would have met some of the amazing people I've made friends with throughout this experience.'

Mostly, loss of confidence was something I heard about from the really high-flying or 'Type A' women, perhaps because they had further to fall. But when I thought about it, women with regular jobs were often going through the same sort of thing; they just expressed it a bit differently. They told me that during the menopausal change they didn't feel like themselves anymore. They described themselves as 'spinny' like a teenager, questioning everything, feeling like their brain didn't belong to them. The term 'brain fog' came up time and time again, and there were many women who had become convinced they had dementia.

There was also a huge amount of anxiety being experienced by midlife women but for many it was difficult to know if it was hormonal or entirely reasonable. We live in anxiety-inducing times after all. The pandemic, climate change, natural disasters, plus screens and devices that make it almost impossible to disconnect from any of it. If you get a rush of anxiety as you're driving along or walking the dog or trying to get to sleep, it hardly seems surprising. Wouldn't it be odd not to feel anxious at times?

The same goes for depression. I've had a bout of it in every decade of my adult life, the worst in my forties. So if my mood is low now is it that same depression back again or is it hormone-driven this time?

According to the North American Menopause Society (NAMS), women have double the rates of depression during the menopause transition and in the years immediately afterwards. NAMS gives the following list as signs of major depression:[4]
- persistent sad, anxious or 'empty' mood
- feelings of hopelessness or pessimism
- irritability
- feelings of guilt, worthlessness or helplessness

And then menopause stole my personality (or at least borrowed it)

- loss of interest or pleasure in hobbies and activities
- decreased energy or fatigue
- moving or talking more slowly
- feeling restless or having trouble sitting still
- difficulty concentrating, remembering or making decisions
- difficulty sleeping, early-morning awakening or oversleeping
- appetite and/or weight changes
- thoughts of death or suicide, or suicide attempts
- aches or pains, headaches, cramps or digestive problems without a clear physical cause and/or that do not ease even with treatment.

It strikes me that this could almost be a list of menopause symptoms. Don't I feel helpless, exhausted, irritated, sleepless and incapable of making a decision on a regular basis? Don't I have unexplained cramps and feelings of pessimism? And the only menopausal women I know who don't have some degree of weight gain are practically nil-by-mouth these days. Given that it's so easy to conflate menopause and depression symptoms, this is a time of life when women need to be nice to themselves. Let's think about emotional wellness rather than mental illness, which is such a huge umbrella term (if depression is an illness, then it's the common cold and most of us will experience it at some stage).

I could do a whole book on depression — possibly I

will at some point. While there is lots of information out there to chew through, there have been a few essential take-out messages I've got from researching the articles I've written over the years.

~

First of all, rightly or wrongly, hormone replacement therapy (HRT) is not the first thing your doctor is going to reach for if you complain about a mood disorder. I spoke to many women who believed that hormones had done wonders to ease their anxiety and crippling depression. They felt calmer and generally much happier. The author Marian Keyes, who has been through major mental health problems, said on the podcast *The Shift* that HRT had helped her and she dreaded the idea that she might have to stop taking it. But there are plenty of women I talked to who hadn't noticed much difference. It was the same with brain fog: for some, hormones brought more clarity, but others said 'Yes I'm on HRT but still don't expect me to remember your birthday'.

For milder depression the first line of defence is always going to be lifestyle tweaks. There is some evidence that switching to a healthier diet can help. Personally, when I feel low all I want to eat are the 'ch' foods — chocolate, cheese and chardonnay. Shopping and cooking healthy meals are efforts I have to force myself to make.

The way of eating with the most good science behind it

is the Mediterranean diet. A version of this diet — which disappointingly has nothing to do with pizza and pasta — has been tested by the Food & Mood Centre at Deakin University in Australia, in what they called the SMILES trial.[5] The researchers wanted to know whether mood improves when diet improves, and lo and behold it did — at least over the 12-week period of the trial. The Mediterranean diet is big on whole grains, vegetables, fruits, legumes, low-fat and unsweetened dairy foods, nuts, fish, lean meats, and olive oil. And it's low on refined carbs, sugar, fried or fast foods and processed meats. Helpfully, you can adapt it to many different cuisines and eating philosophies. There is also an interesting 2019 Japanese observational study[6] that shows increasing your intake of vitamin B_6 and oily fish can help reduce the severity of hot flushes.

It makes sense that having a healthy microbiome — the colony of bacteria in your gut — is going to mean having a happier brain, as the two body parts are connected through millions of nerves (most importantly the vagus nerve) and are constantly communicating back and forth. Also, much of the body's supply of the mood-regulating hormone serotonin is manufactured by bacteria in the gut. However, many mood-challenged women I talked to were big on nutrition, so an extra handful of walnuts and a lot more salmon were unlikely to make a noticeable difference.

~

Being active is another natural mood-enhancer. It promotes the release of endorphins, a group of chemicals produced by our nervous system and pituitary gland that induce a feeling of wellbeing. They also boost our levels of serotonin and another feel-good brain chemical called dopamine, and balance our levels of the stress hormone adrenaline.

Outdoor activity is especially helpful. Being surrounded by plants and trees has been found to promote lower concentrations of the stress hormone cortisol, lower blood pressure and increase feelings of vitality. One study showed that spending 120 minutes in nature each week was associated with good health and wellbeing;[7] and in Japan, where *shinrin-yoku* — or forest bathing — is part of the national public health programme, people are encouraged to get out on to designated therapy trails.

The science shows that we get the biggest boost to our wellbeing if we can be mindful while we're amidst nature, so that means turning off our phones, removing our headphones and really noticing the birdsong and smells, the patterns of nature and the colours. If we can bring ourselves to be more present, that seems to boost the boost.

Meditation and mindfulness can stabilise mood, as can getting out of the house and connecting with friends. It's called behavioural activation and there are a host of options, but they all require one key thing — motivation. The problem is that when you're feeling terrible, the last thing you want to do is leave the house to socialise or exercise. You might much rather stay in bed or on the sofa bingeing Netflix and subsisting on the garnishes from cocktails (olives in martinis, orange in negronis, celery in a Bloody Mary, cucumber in Pimm's . . . it's more varied than you might think, but still not recommended; trust me, I've tried it).

For behavioural activation to work, you have to do the opposite of what your brain is telling you to do. And if you're severely depressed, that's not going to happen.

~

In my forties I wasted an entire year trying to pull myself together. It was a year of my life where I cried all the time and felt completely stuck in a job that didn't suit me (I was quite good at the job, but it wasn't good for *me*). The reason I didn't ask for help sooner was that I felt ashamed. I had good friends, a lovely husband, a perfectly nice house and enough money to live on, so I didn't think I had any right to feel the way I did. Finally I went to the doctor, burst into tears and told her that my life felt like a great big mountain I couldn't climb, and she hastily wrote a prescription for fluoxetine (the anti-depressant drug sold under the brand name Prozac).

Anti-depressants aren't effective for everyone — about a third of people get no benefit, and potentially these drugs are even less effective for menopause-related depression. Geneticists are still trying to work out why one individual might respond to a drug like fluoxetine that boosts serotonin, while someone else does better on a medication that gets different parts of the brain talking to each other. Some psychedelic drugs like MDMA and ketamine are being investigated for hard-to-treat depression — but not specifically, as far as I know, for hormone-driven disorders.

Pre-menopausal at the time (I think!), I was fortunate that the first anti-depressant I tried worked for me. I remember one evening cooking dinner while chatting to my husband, and thinking 'Oh, this is nice' — then being shocked to realise that it was a long time since I'd enjoyed anything at all.

So don't be like me. Get help sooner. Ask your doctor if anti-depressants might work; sign up for talk-therapy if it's available; download one of the mental wellbeing apps (John Kirwan has a free one called Mentemia) — and tell your whānau what is going on, as most family and friends will want to support you. The thing with serious depression is that when you are tight in its grip, it's difficult to imagine ever feeling better. But I've been depressed. And then I've felt better. So if it happens again, I'll hold onto that knowledge — that it will get better. If it's happening to you right now, please know that you won't be in that dark place forever. It may take some trial and error, but you'll find the thing — or combination of things — that works for you;

and while in the future you may have to be more careful with your emotional wellbeing, and take a few preventative measures, that's not as hard as it may seem when you're deep in the pits of it.

I came across the following from the author Matt Haig — who as well as writing wonderful novels has been very open about his own mental health struggles — and I think it's hopeful and useful. What Matt tweeted on 17 June 2021 was this:

21 years ago this summer I nearly died by suicide because I knew I'd never be happy again. Today I put away the dishes then stood in the garden and let summer rain soak me to my skin. I felt so alive and quietly euphoric I wanted to reach back through time to tell me I was wrong.

A year after that consultation with my doctor, with my mood stabilised and having ditched the job I shouldn't have been doing, I weaned myself off the anti-depressants. Since then I've got smarter at identifying the things that can trigger depression in me. If I over-face myself by taking on too much — trying to write a second novel while editing a weekly magazine, for instance — then I start to slide. Learning to say no and take the pressure off before my mental health declines is a work in progress and isn't always possible, but I'm trying. I don't want to go back to that blackness, so I watch over myself.

This has got trickier since my hormones went haywire. One day I might feel entirely fine and capable, then the next I'll be overwhelmed and not coping. All I can do is brace myself and hang on, knowing that no mood lasts forever. It's a wild ride, yes, but it's some comfort to know that other women are on it, too. So many of the smart, inspirational women I spoke to during the research for this book — women who seemed to have all their shit together — shared similar thoughts and feelings. They were all hanging on during that wild ride, too.

~

We spend over a third of our lives being post-menopausal, but on the way there relationships can end and careers flounder. Some of us might actually need to get out of that job or that relationship, and looking back they will be glad that the hormonal shift was what prompted them to do it. But my husband is one of the good ones, and I'm glad we stuck it out through my swingiest moods and hottest flushes and fiercest rages, even if I wasn't always easy to live with and he wasn't always great at dealing with that.

And then menopause stole my personality (or at least borrowed it)

It's been over a year since my last period so I'm officially post-menopause. The rages have subsided and I don't cry quite so readily. I still have days when I don't know whether I can manage any of the things I ought to be capable of. Or when I go to the supermarket for salad ingredients and emerge with five kinds of chocolate. And I do still have those random attacks of anxiety. But I feel more like me now, and less like an imposter.

The good news is that at some point the menopause gives us our personalities back. We may even end up as better versions of our original selves. Less emotional, more even, energetic and confident, too — not hostage anymore to the monthly cycling of our hormones, but out the other side and free of it all. Isn't that something to look forward to?

'Imagine your future self walking on the path ahead of you. Let her lead you.'

— *Gloria Steinem,* The Truth Will Set You Free, But First It Will Piss You Off!

Chapter 5

And then the menopause (hopefully) borrowed my libido

My husband and I were out for a walk one day and saw a sign in the window of a local shop that read: 'Closed for business'. When I told him I might have those very words tattooed over my vagina, my husband didn't laugh. I was only half joking, and he didn't find it funny at all.

As previously mentioned, I like the man I'm married

to. I enjoy hanging out with him and miss him if he's not around. After almost 30 years together, I even still fancy him. But at some point in my mid-fifties my libido went missing.

It makes evolutionary sense that I no longer need the sexual drive I once had. I'm not useful for propagating the species anymore, and so sex isn't necessary. Still, it had never occurred to me that the urge would just disappear one day, as if a tap had been switched off. It felt like I had lost something very essential.

I want to want sex. For a start, I have a husband and it seems a waste not to take advantage of that. I also had a life-plan for if he left me in the next decade or so, and that involved taking lots of late-life lovers. This was inspired by a really interesting memoir I read, *A Round-Heeled Woman* by Jane Juska, who did just that. I quite liked the idea of being a sexagenarian strumpet should I find myself unwillingly single. But now I was high and dry — literally drier, as it turns out.

I had noticed that I had become as dry as a chip in other areas, too. My skin requires constant moisturising, my hair guzzles conditioner and oils, my fingernails snap, and even my eyes demand the constant application of hydrating drops and sessions with warm compresses to get some natural oils flowing.

Was my vagina also drying out? I tried not to think about it. Generally it has been down there for years doing its own thing with very little interference aside from a daily cleanse, a regular Pap smear, a lot of tampons back in the day and the occasional visit from a penis. It wasn't prone to getting fat, nothing needed trimming (the bush is back!), it never got photographed, and it seemed like the one part of me that I didn't have to worry about too much. But for the purposes of this book I did a little investigation, and indeed there did seem to be some changes in the old-lady garden. 'Moist' is an off-putting word, but it's even more off-putting to realise that you're a little less moist than you used to be.

~

Associate professor Helen Roberts, an endocrinologist who works at the menopause clinic at Auckland's Greenlane Hospital, told me that vaginal dryness is often something that comes along later, a kind of parting gesture of the menopause transition (my words, not hers) that affects women in their later fifties.

It's one of those things we *really* don't want to talk about and we *really* ought to because a solution is very available. There is a cream called Ovestin that contains oestriol, a minor female sex hormone. The prevailing wisdom is that it's a very safe product for most to use.

If you read Medsafe's data sheet on it then you might be scared off, but the dosage is low and all the doctors I spoke to recommended Ovestin cream as an effective way to treat vaginal dryness. Also, the Australasian Menopause Society states that there is no risk of breast cancer with vaginal oestrogen. I did ask Medsafe, why the confusion? The response was that the information on their data sheet comes from the pharmaceutical company responsible for the product. For it to change, the company would need to apply to Medsafe and provide data and evidence demonstrating that the warning could be removed. Medsafe would then assess that data against internationally agreed standards. That might take a while, then! This also provides an example of how difficult it is, even for health professionals, to establish what is harmful and what is beneficial when it comes to hormone therapies.

Those women I spoke to who were using Ovestin said it made all the difference, even if it could be a bit messy. Some had struggled on for ages before realising that something very simple could be done to improve their moistness (ugh). Many were very eager that other women should hear about it, and not suffer the way they had themselves.

The official term for midlife problems in the down-below area is 'genito-urinary syndrome of the menopause (GSM)'. This is a bit of a mouthful, but a vast improvement on previous terms such as vaginal atrophy ('atrophy' is a far more off-putting word than 'moist').

An international survey[1] showed that post-menopausal

woman have a low understanding of GSM. And while around 70% of midlife women have symptoms, only 7% get treatment. It seems that we're not asking for help because it's embarrassing. I've been told that wāhine Māori consider the vagina tapu (sacred) and feel whakamā (shyness) about it, and I'm quite sure that this is an attitude shared by women across other cultures. While it's understandable, I think it's unhelpful for our health and wellbeing — which is why I'm being so dazzlingly open about my own. It's just a vagina, designed for things to enter and emerge from; a very useful part of the body that we shouldn't be shy of mentioning to a medical professional if necessary.

Undesirable dryness isn't the only problem we menopausal women are having down there. There are oestrogen receptors in the vagina, urethra, bladder and pelvic floor. So all these areas can be affected by a lack of the hormone during the peri-menopause and menopause.

Some women have burning and itching down below. Sex is painful and they might bleed afterwards. They may also have pain riding a bicycle or a horse — or even just sitting down. This is because along with the decreased moisture there may also come reduced elasticity and collagen, so the tissue there is more fragile and easily injured. Basically, if it's happening to the skin on the outside of your body, it's probably also happening to the epithelial (surface) layer inside your vulva and vagina.

And wait, there's more. Muscles in your previously efficient peeing system are atrophying (ugh), so you may need to pee more often and more urgently. And as the pH level (which measures how acid or alkaline something is) of the vagina changes, becoming more alkaline, some women will experience recurrent urinary tract infections. You don't need to be sexually active to not want any of that.

Some women are at higher risk of GSM — if you've had certain cancer treatments or take various medications — and that is another reason why we really need to talk to our doctors about this. There can be a lot to get through in a 15-minute GP consultation and if you don't bring it up, they might not.

HRT can help, but doesn't in all cases; and you may choose not to take it (more on that later). Even so, I believe you should consider using an oestrogen cream or pessaries to restore the health of your vagina. New Zealand's drug-buying agency Pharmac tends to fund one option in each category of drugs. So for GSM, your option is Ovestin. Endocrinologist Anna Fenton says if things have been drying out down there for a while, it can sting when you start putting a really active cream in your vagina so she advises starting gently and slowly. And actually, it's preferable not to wait until things get dire, because, unlike hot flushes, GSM generally doesn't go away by itself. The smart move is to start treatment earlier and prevent future problems.

~

It may take a while to notice a change after you start using Ovestin, and there are other things you can do to boost its benefits. Most of this is good advice for general vaginal health. So no shaving or waxing of the genital area (like I said, the bush is back). Avoid using scented products, including loo paper. Limit time spent in tight-fitting underwear, wet togs and sweaty trackies. Wear cotton knickers, except in bed when you should let your vagina get some air. Don't douche (personally I'm not sure why you'd want to, but the evidence seems to be that there are no benefits and a considerable chance of harm). Your vagina doesn't need to be purged — it has its own colony of natural bacteria and you don't want to upset them. A splash of warm water and a gentle pat dry should be sufficient. If you must use soap, make it a mild one and rinse carefully.

If you're itchy, then the Australasian Menopause Society suggests cool washes using a dilute solution of bicarbonate of soda a.k.a. baking soda (½ teaspoon in 1 litre of water) and says that applying natural sweet almond and avocado oils can help, as can vitamin E cream — choose one especially designed for vaginal use. Also be aware that oils can damage the integrity of latex, so shouldn't be used alongside condoms. For the same reason, water-based lubes should be used for more comfortable and enjoyable sex (I know — it's like your vagina suddenly needs its own bathroom cabinet).

I did get sent a pot of a New Zealand-made product, NatFem Balm, which is a blend of natural botanicals like coconut oil and calendula, designed for vaginal dryness. I may give it a go if I get around to having sex before its use-by date. But I seem to spend my entire life smearing a natural botanical balm on my lips and they're still dry, so while it's worth a try if Ovestin doesn't appeal, I'm not holding out huge hope.

Another option out there is vaginal rejuvenation using a fractional carbon-dioxide laser. There is a treatment called the Mona Lisa Touch available in New Zealand. Lasering has been around as a facial beauty treatment for some time and this one works on the same principle. It creates pinpoint burns, and as the body kicks in with the healing process it plumps up the vagina.

Considering how much it hurt when I had some brown sun-spots lasered off my face, the thought of putting my vagina through it isn't appealing, but the claim from those offering the treatment is that it's pain-free and endocrinologist Anna Fenton says that's what she hears from the patients who've tried it. Does it work? We've been in a limbo-land, with some health professionals enthusiastic about it and others advising a more careful approach. For Anna, vaginal laser therapy has been something to consider only when women were having major difficulties tolerating

Ovestin. Her concern was reports about burns and scarring, increased pain with sex and narrowing of the urethra making peeing more difficult. Plus there was no real guidance on how often the treatment should be repeated or whether it should be repeated at all. Now the latest research out of Australia isn't encouraging. A randomised clinical trial[2] has found that laser treatment isn't any more effective than a placebo at improving vaginal menopause symptoms and the researchers have advised women not to bother.

~

Having said all that about the vagina, I actually don't believe that my libido fled simply because of the state of mine. There must be some other reason it broke up with me, but it's difficult to pinpoint exactly what. The thing about sex is that if you're tired, hot, grumpy, stressed, anxious or a bit depressed then it's not exactly a turn-on, and I'm often a little bit of all those things. And really, who cares *what* caused my libido to leave? The question really is where did it go and how can I get it back?

A whole industry exists around products that promise to enhance sexual satisfaction. Most of them are designed to increase blood flow to the genital area to help men get an erection — like Viagra (generic name sildenafil). Female versions of these products are being developed by drug companies. In 2019 the FDA in the US approved Vyleesi, a medication that comes in a push-pen device for injection. It was found to increase desire in a proportion of women, but it also made a lot of them feel nauseous — which is not how I like to get in the mood. A daily pill designed to increase women's sex drive was similarly plagued with unsexy side-effects.

At age 70, actress Jane Fonda spoke out about using testosterone to boost her libido. There have been years of debate among experts over the wisdom of this therapy for women. Although generally thought of as a male hormone, testosterone is produced naturally in women's bodies by the ovaries and adrenal glands — albeit in far smaller amounts — and it also supports bone strength, muscle strength, energy levels and self-confidence. As we age, decade by decade, our testosterone levels drop. The big question is whether there is any benefit in replacing the lost hormone.

In 2019 the International Menopause Society released a position statement[3] on the use of testosterone to boost libido. This followed research by Australian endocrinologist Susan Davis, who has found that it has a clear benefit for the sexual wellbeing of some women post-menopause. While it doesn't help any of the other symptoms, like general wellbeing and mood, testosterone treatment can improve desire, pleasure, arousal and orgasm in post-menopausal women who are experiencing problems. I interviewed Susan Davis at the time; her view was that we want to continue to be sexually active for longer nowadays, so while she wasn't advocating dosing everyone up on testosterone, we have to at least give women the choice.

One issue has been that everything to do with testosterone has been designed for men. But there is now a testosterone cream designed specifically for women, AndroFeme, developed in Australia and available here on prescription. At the time of writing, there is only one supplier in the whole of New Zealand, Bays Health Pharmacy on Auckland's North Shore (meanwhile, the little blue Viagra pills that help so many men with their erection problems are available in every pharmacy in the land).

Jane Fonda gave up on testosterone because it gave her acne. Weight gain and excessive body or facial hair are other potential side-effects, although in her research Susan Davis found these weren't serious enough to put women off taking it.

Be aware that too much testosterone is harmful for women, causing anything from acne, to a permanently lowered voice. So a low dose is crucial, and careful monitoring is advised to be sure the levels are in the normal range and the treatment is providing enough benefit, especially initially.

All of the endocrinologists I spoke to said that

testosterone wouldn't be the first thing they would reach for to help a woman's flagging libido. First they would try to improve sleep and make sure there was no vaginal discomfort. It's not that they're being obstructive, refusing to give patients the treatment they ask for, but more that there isn't yet enough information about long-term safety and doctors tend to be cautious.

Another androgen (androgens are hormones usually thought of as male, but are also produced in women in smaller amounts) that gets touted as a libido booster for women is DHEA. Overseas this is available in gel form for vaginal dryness, but there's no evidence that giving it to post-menopausal women helps them get their groove back.

~

Endocrinologist Anna Fenton says that the drop in sex drive is a really big issue for menopausal women, and is something she always asks patients about because it's not a topic they will usually bring up themselves the first time they meet her.

'The best evidence we have is that life probably has more influence on libido than hormones do,' she says.

With that in mind, I'm planning to test a new approach. At the risk of sounding like a 1950s marriage manual, I'm trying to make more effort. I've decided that sex is a little like going to a spin class — I might not necessarily feel like doing it right at that moment, but once I get going I enjoy it and feel great afterwards. It's about having the time, opportunity and not being so knackered that you fall asleep the moment you get horizontal (sex, not spin).

Not every woman I spoke to had bothered going looking for their lost libido. Some thought that there were upsides to not being bothered by it.

'After menopause you're all vigour and vim, you're not ruled by your vagina,' one woman told me, apparently relishing the chance to expend her energy on other things.

Another said, more wistfully but with acceptance, 'Sex was a long silvery river that had run through my life and then came to an end.'

There may be lots of couples out there living in platonic bliss, but for me it seems like a necessary part of having a relationship — not a daily part, not necessarily even weekly, but still necessary. So while the lady garden may require a little irrigation, I'm not going to have 'closed for business' tattooed over it anytime soon.

Suzanne Paul

'I've got to the age where I know what I want.'

If you've watched TV in New Zealand over the past 25 years, you'll know who Suzanne Paul is (although she's probably still most famous for selling a bronzing product with the catchphrase 'thousands of luminous spheres'). Suzanne's in her mid-sixties now and not such a familiar face on television, as women presenters tend to get shipped off our screens when they get older — even if, like Suzanne, they put in the maintenance to stay looking great.

Suzanne had a full-on menopause — she bloated, she sweated, her moods swung around — and it coincided with a period of grief in her life, which was a whole extra layer of tough for a woman who knew herself as a positive, resilient person. Also, although Suzanne took a while to realise it, she was suffering from GSM.

'For several months I thought I had cystitis,' she says. 'I kept going to the pharmacy and getting the sachets for it [potassium or sodium citrate cystitis sachets reduce the acidity of your urine and lessen the burning sensation when urinating]. Then I started worrying because I was desperate to go to the loo all the time — on planes I'd have to ask for an aisle seat.'

Eventually she talked to her doctor, who asked if she still wanted to have sex. When Suzanne said yes, actually she did, she was prescribed Ovestin.

Suzanne has since met other women who have had a similar experience of not understanding the cause of their symptoms and not being aware that oestrogen cream could fix it — but, as she says, you don't know what you don't know.

Ovestin was the only form of hormone therapy Suzanne used, but if she'd known what lay ahead when peri-menopause arrived she might have asked for more help.

'Bloating . . . that was the bane of my life,' she says. 'I looked like I was nine months pregnant, little stick-like arms and legs with a big stomach poking out. You can't eat like you used to. Your diet gets narrower and narrower. And the night sweats were a killer. I'd wake every night with my head boiling. If I had a nightie on, it had to come right off. And then my temperature would come down and I'd be freezing and have to put on another nightie. I was getting no sleep and was exhausted with this continual hot flushing.'

She still gets flushes now, but not like she used to, and has learned to recognise that one is coming on as a few moments before she has an odd feeling in her stomach, as if she is ravenously hungry.

There have been other health issues potentially linked to menopause. Suzanne has developed tinnitus and aching joints in her fingers. But thanks to 'tweakments' like Botox and fillers she looks youthful, and is prepared to have more in the future because looking good is important to her.

On the inside, in her head specifically, things are probably better than ever. 'I've got to the age where I know what I want, I know how to get it and I'm going to do it,' she says.

When her marriage ended, she started looking for love again and had a list of attributes her ideal man would have. Her new partner Patrick ticks so many of those boxes that she says it's almost like she 'magicked him up'.

When I talked to Suzanne she was about to leap into a new phase of her life, with plans to start a business, build a house and get married to lovely, handsome, funny Patrick, who never loses his temper and is always laughing. And yes, she's still using that oestrogen cream.

Chapter 6

And then the menopause destroyed my superpower

Often I find myself wishing that I could plug myself in like an iPhone to get charged up with energy. None of the other ways of powering up seem to be working for me anymore. I'M SO TIRED. Those were three words I heard from so many women once we started talking about this stage of life. Some were juggling ridiculously busy lives — but what they'd been dealing with before, now seemed too hard. And there was an obvious reason for this outbreak of fatigue. Nobody was sleeping.

'We may as well all call each other at 3 a.m. for a chat because we're all awake,' said one of the exhausted.

Sleeping used to be my superpower. I was a genius at it. At around 10.30 p.m. I'd fall into bed, then drift off straight away and not wake until my alarm went off at 7 a.m. Generally, when I heard it ringing my first thought was that I couldn't wait until the moment when I would be able to dive back under the covers again.

It's almost as if I've been reprogrammed now, because in midlife none of that is true anymore. My superpower has left me. Bed is no longer my favourite place.

There are times when I can't get to sleep at all. There's the 3 a.m. wake-up with my heart pounding and my head full of panic and dread. Possibly even worse are the periods of living like a breakfast radio host — waking at 4.30 a.m. knowing that I'm never going to get back to sleep and may as well get up. I wrote a large portion of a novel at that hour. When I went back to review the 'insomnia chapters' I thought they might be the work of a madwoman — but no, they were fine, which only shows how wide awake I must have been.

Please do NOT talk to me about sleep hygiene. I've read all those articles about having a properly dark bedroom, staying off screens and using the bed only for sleeping and sex. I may have even written some of them, and for that I apologise because what I know now is that you can do absolutely everything right and *still* not sleep. Or, conversely, you can do everything wrong and yet for some reason have a good night's rest.

~

Insomnia is a boringly common menopause symptom, and the conventional wisdom has been that it's linked to sweaty hot flushes — so if you can fix them then you'll fix sleep. Like pretty much everything, though, it's much more complex than that.

For midlife women, sleeplessness tends to be caused by a perfect storm. For a start, melatonin (a hormone that's vital for sleep) decreases with age. We also have higher levels of the 'stress hormone' cortisol, which is essential to kick-start us in the morning but unhelpful if it decides to spike at night. Then there are brain chemicals called orexins (also known as hypocretins) that stimulate wakefulness, and it seems that in menopause we have higher levels of these in our blood.

Add in a few other issues. Perhaps you have sleep apnoea (a potentially serious sleep disorder in which breathing repeatedly stops and starts). Restless legs syndrome. Aching joints that keep you awake once you do wake up. You're struggling with a lot of stress. And you need to go to the loo a lot more. Once you start adding everything up, it's amazing that any of us is getting a wink of sleep.

Here's the real horror story — not sleeping is appalling

for your health. During deep sleep, your body manufactures and releases cytokines — the warriors of the immune system — as well as killer T-cells and antibodies. So if you are sleep-deprived, you are more likely to get sick.

In one study,[1] led by a San Francisco sleep researcher called Aric Prather, they got 164 healthy people to wear monitors to assess their sleep. Then they brought them into the lab, squirted the common cold virus up their noses and monitored them. Those who slept for fewer than six hours were four times more likely to develop a cold than those who got seven or more hours of sleep, despite the virus being exactly the same. Sleep was more important than any other factor in predicting each person's likelihood of catching a cold, regardless of how old they were, their education or income, or even if they were a smoker.

The impact on the immune system is one of the main reasons why people who sleep badly tend to die younger. There are plenty of other motivations to rest well, of course:
-    While we're in deep sleep a network of channels in the brain, known as the glymphatic system, opens up and lets cerebrospinal fluid flow through the brain tissue and wash away potentially neurotoxic waste products. As we age we tend to get less deep sleep, so become less efficient at clearing away these waste proteins, and that is believed to be one of the drivers of dementia — former UK prime minister

Margaret Thatcher, who famously got by on four hours of sleep a night, experienced steep cognitive decline later in life.

- Stress hormones are lower when we sleep more. Deep sleep is also when the brain sorts through its memories and shifts the useful ones into storage, which might explain the failing memory of old age. And it is also when we subconsciously process our emotions.

- Sleeping for less than five hours a night has been associated with weaker bones and a higher chance of osteoporosis.

- If you don't sleep well, it affects your body's ability to control blood sugar levels. Over time, this is associated with diabetes, high blood pressure and cardiovascular disease. Being deprived of sleep also alters your appetite hormones so you tend to eat more, then you gain weight, which also ups your risk of diabetes. It's all so interlinked that it's dizzying.

- Some of us are genetically bad sleepers, so that adds an extra layer of complication.

To function at our very best we need four to five sleep cycles that are comprised of the deep and restorative non-REM sleep, the lighter, dream-filled REM sleep, and a stage known as stable light sleep. These cycles are 90 minutes long on average, but vary across the night. So we get more very deep sleep earlier and a predominance of REM sleep towards the end. The old adage that every hour of sleep before midnight is worth two after midnight turns out to be rubbish. We need all the sleep cycles, and that means seven to eight hours of rest time to fit them all in.

Of course, none of this is any help at all if you want to sleep but can't. It's probably just making you feel worse (sorry).

During prolonged periods of insomnia I can feel quite manic. Mostly, though, I'm exhausted and feel like I can't deal with any of the things I'm meant to be doing. It's a bone-deep, paralysing, swimming-through-syrup fatigue. That's when the brain fog and the forgetfulness strike. Also the low moods and wanting to cry, and being on a shorter fuse than usual with other people.

~

Sleeplessness is one of the main reasons the women I spoke with gave for taking HRT. Many said it helped, but it wasn't a miracle for all of them. This is probably because the brain adapts to a pattern of not sleeping and it's difficult to break the habit. A re-set is required.

There is a whole suite of things you can do, but going to the doctor for sleeping pills probably isn't one of them. While drugs can help in the short term, there's pretty good evidence that long-term they don't improve disturbed sleep for midlife women.[2] Medsafe recommends, for example, that zopiclone (brand name Imovane) be used only for a maximum of four weeks. Hypno-sedatives increase brain fog, they put older people at greater risk of falls, and you can become dependent on them. Also, your body builds up tolerance over time so you have to move on to something stronger.

There are drug-free approaches that are more likely to have a lasting effect.

Alex Bartle is the director of a national network of Sleep Well Clinics in New Zealand. He says that many people make the mistake of focusing on the *amount* of sleep they are getting, when *quality* is just as important. Rather than going to bed early and then tossing and turning, Alex advises sleep restriction. It seems counter-intuitive, particularly if you're exhausted and longing to go to bed early, but the idea is that over time you increase sleep efficiency.

Sleep restriction involves spending less time in bed and ensuring that when you are there you are resting properly. The first step is to note the percentage of time in bed that you are actually sleeping. A wearable sleep tracker that measures heart rate is one way to do this, but if you don't have one then you can still keep a sleep diary. Record how well you slept, what your mood is like, whether you drank coffee or alcohol (and when), when you ate your last meal of the day, whether you exercised, etc., so you can see exactly what is going on.

If you've learned from your self-tracking that you are only getting six hours of sleep a night, then you should go to bed later — say at 1 a.m. if you plan to wake at 7 a.m. The rules are that you never cut down the time in bed to less than five hours, don't snooze during the day, and stick to the routine rigorously. As you stop associating bed with stress and worry, and as your sleep efficiency improves, you can keep moving your bedtime 20 minutes earlier until you're in a normal routine. It may take a while for this approach to work, so keep at it for a few weeks.

~

When you're lying awake, head buzzing with thoughts and feeling anxious, it's better to get up for a while so that bed doesn't become a place that you associate with anxiety.

Before the Industrial Revolution it was normal for people to sleep in two blocks. They went to bed when it got dark, slept for five hours, woke up and did a bit of reading or had sex, then went back for a second stint of sleep. The idea that we should zonk out for a consecutive seven or eight hours is relatively new, and if you can make a bi-phasic sleep pattern work for you then why try to fight it? Keep the gap to an hour or less, and do something fairly boring in it. Calm the mind with meditation or by journalling (writing down worries and feelings) or listening to soothing music. Reading a really dull book is good too (so not one of mine!).

Also important is getting outdoors every morning so that you wake up properly. Light suppresses the sleep hormone melatonin and triggers the release of the good-mood hormone serotonin. This happens when the light hits your retina, so wearing sunglasses will block the effect.

At night we need to behave the opposite way, avoiding light sources like phones and tablets as they delay the natural production of melatonin — which is converted from serotonin by the pineal gland in the brain — and decrease feelings of sleeplessness. Apparently even wearing lenses that block blue light, or having our devices switched to dark mode, can still interfere with sleep, and that's believed to be due to the interactive nature of screens and the fact that we hold them close to our face.

If your ageing pineal gland is on a go-slow with melatonin production, you can take an oral version to boost levels of the hormone. Melatonin supplements are available in New Zealand on prescription from a doctor, or if you're over 55 you can get it direct from a registered pharmacist for up to 13 weeks. It's not funded (but zopiclone, with all its downsides, is — go figure), so not only is it more expensive but the dose is lower than you'll find in many of the supplements available on overseas websites.

The Ministry of Health says that it is illegal to import a

prescription medicine into New Zealand unless you have provided Medsafe with a prescription or a letter from your doctor, and then you're allowed a maximum of three months' supply. The Medsafe website specifically mentions melatonin. Obviously I'm not going to encourage you to do anything illicit. I'm just putting it out there that many women I spoke to were scoring slow-release melatonin over the internet and said they wouldn't be without it.

Melatonin tends to be prescribed more as a re-set for people travelling across time zones. It's not completely without side-effects — some people experience headaches, stomach cramps and dizziness — and you're not meant to mix it with alcohol.

Alex Bartle of the Sleep Well Clinic reckons that while it is relatively safe, melatonin's effect is mainly psychological. Personally I'm pretty sure that taking modified-release melatonin is beneficial. It helps me fall asleep more quickly, and if I wake during the night I don't lie there tossing and turning but drift off again more easily. In my experience, getting a decent night's sleep makes everything else seem better. However, I'm unconvinced that taking a short course of melatonin will re-set sleep habits for good. If my body isn't producing effective amounts of melatonin naturally anymore, then surely, like any other hormone, it's necessary to take it on an ongoing basis?

Melatonin doesn't knock you out like a sedative does. Instead it prepares your body naturally for sleep, making you feel drowsier and calm, so the idea is to take it half an hour before bed and then do something relaxing. Whether the hormone is entirely safe for long-term use is still in question, but it seems highly likely that it is a whole lot better than not getting any sleep at all.

As for other supplements, well, the shelves of pharmacies and health stores are loaded with stuff to help us sleep, because it's obviously big business. My suggestion would be to try some of the lower-priced options first.

The nutrient magnesium plays an important role in the nervous system. Among its many tasks is regulating melatonin, and it also binds to a neurotransmitter, GABA, which is responsible for calming down brain activity. It's easy to find this essential mineral in the foods we eat, even if you're strictly plant-based — it's in seeds, nuts, pulses and leafy greens, for example. Most of us eat lots of those things, right? The question is whether taking extra magnesium helps you sleep if you're not deficient in it in the first place. There's a lack of hard-core science on this (most of the research seems to have been done with elderly people), but I'd say it's worth a try since a bit of extra magnesium isn't going to do any harm or cost a lot.

The amino acids glycine and tyrine are also commonly used to calm the nervous system and promote sleep. Both are safe and affordable, and so are up there with magnesium at the top of the sleep-boosting shopping list.

There are loads of other options. Some people swear by tart cherry juice, others prefer calming herbs like passionflower, valerian and skullcap. There's probably going to be some trial and error required to find out what suits you. Many pharmaceutical medicines aren't effective for every single person (remember that statistic about antidepressants not working for a third of people), so surely the same would be true of natural medicines? Just give them a fair go and take any natural therapy that you're experimenting with for a few weeks to give it a chance — so long as there aren't any adverse effects, obviously.

~

Sleeplessness can actually be as much about what you *don't* put into your body as what you do. In menopause, things you got on well with for years suddenly aren't your friends anymore — and that can be hard to take. I'm struggling to break up with coffee and wine because we've been together for a long time. But caffeine is a stimulant, and there's evidence to prove that drinking it as much as six hours before bedtime disrupts sleep.[3] Also, as we get older our bodies metabolise caffeine more slowly so it takes longer to leave our system. Having a coffee close to bedtime won't necessarily stop you dropping off, but it does interfere with deep sleep.

As for wine, while I valiantly battle on and keep drinking, the science is pretty clear that as a midlife woman I shouldn't. Our biology changes as we age. The liver progressively shrinks, the total amount of fluid in the body decreases and the enzymes that metabolise alcohol diminish, meaning that it stays in our system for longer. This applies whatever your gender, but women do it tougher due to generally having a smaller body size and lower amounts of those critical enzymes in the first place.

The other problem with alcohol is that it keeps the liver busy. If the body's main detoxification system is focused on eliminating introduced toxins like alcohol, it neglects other jobs such as breaking down oestrogen.

'If we keep drinking each day, the hormone starts to build up and we become oestrogen-dominant,' explains holistic nutritionist Jessica Giljam-Brown. 'That's where all those problems around peri-menopause come in, like weight gain, mood changes and difficult menstrual periods.'

The impact on oestrogen is behind the increased risk of some breast cancers for women drinkers. And while there isn't much firm evidence around hot flushes, I'm pretty sure it doesn't improve them at all.

Alcohol is a sedative so it may help you fall asleep more quickly, but that sedative effect wears off and it has a disrupting effect on the rest of the night as the body works to metabolise it. Waking up with your heart juddering at 3 a.m.? That's the chardonnay you enjoyed a little earlier coming back to haunt you.

Ironically, women are being targeted by the alcohol industry, which isn't slow to spot a potential market. There's a growing range of Instagram-friendly pink beers, ciders and wines, and if you keep an eye out you'll notice girly-pink drinks being spruiked in female-friendly spaces, often in quite creative ways. Then there are the often-funny Mummy Wine Culture memes you'll come across on social media platforms: 'The most expensive part of having kids is all the wine you have to drink' or 'Wine is to women what duct tape is to men — it fixes everything'. There are Facebook communities with names like Mummy Needs A Wine and Mommy Needs A Vodka. There are T-shirts, mugs, coasters. There's no knowing where all this content originates from, but growing #dontpinkmydrink and Living Sober movements are providing some push-back.

Personally, I don't think that a couple of glasses of wine in an evening is the deal-breaker for me when it comes to sleep. What I *eat* can make more of a difference to my menopausal digestive system. Spicy and rich foods keep me awake these days, as do members of the allium family — onions, leeks and garlic. And I have definitely broken up with Jerusalem artichokes. The last time we met I was so gassy afterwards that even the dog wouldn't sleep with me. Epic farting is not conducive to restful slumber, I find. Or to anything else.

When you eat also makes a difference. Dr Satchin Panda of the Salk Institute, a leading expert on circadian rhythms, advises finishing the last meal of the day at least three hours before bedtime. This is because eating raises your core temperature, which naturally falls as bedtime approaches, triggering sleep. It cranks up your digestive system, and if you eat late then your pancreas has to spew out insulin at a time when all of that should be slowing down.

~

Rather than enjoying a late-night snack, the time before bed will ideally be spent unwinding. Mindfulness and meditation can be really useful as relaxation aids, although they don't work for everybody and they're not necessarily something you pick up easily and quickly.

A very simple mindfulness exercise is to sit and focus your thoughts on your breath. As those thoughts wander, let them drift away then bring your attention back to breathing in and out.

If you're a physical person then progressive muscle relaxation might suit you more and is only marginally more complex. Again, breath is the key. While inhaling, contract one muscle group — say clench a fist with your right hand — then relax it on the exhale. Take a 10- to 20-second break before progressing through all the other muscle groups — forearms, upper arms, belly, thigh, etc. It might not necessarily make you fall asleep straight away, but it can help to relax you.

If you're using a technique that everyone else says is wonderful and it doesn't solve your problems, that can create a negative feedback loop — 'What's wrong with me? Why can't I do this?' — which might actually make you feel worse. Like most things, trying it and giving it some time is the best you can do. Any approach will only work for a percentage of people, and that might not include you.

The same goes for cognitive behavioural therapy (CBT). This can supply some useful strategies to get you through the potentially low moods and anxieties of the menopause transition, and even help ease hot flushes, but it isn't a fix-all for everyone.

Slow diaphragmatic breathing is one technique worth borrowing, as you can do it anytime, anywhere. Ideally you'll be sitting in a chair or lying on your bed. Relax your shoulders, put your hands on your stomach and take a slow breath in through your nose — your stomach should expand as your lungs fill up. Then exhale slowly through your mouth. It's not about taking huge breaths — just normal ones but at a slower pace — and it's important that you're breathing deep into your stomach rather than in a shallow way, from your chest. Do this for ten minutes, ideally twice a day. Making one of those times prior to bed might be a good idea, although staying on top of tension throughout our waking hours is likely to improve our sleeping ones.

Also remember another old adage: 'The time to relax is when you don't have time for it.' That one turns out to be *completely* true.

~

All this is just the tip of the sleep iceberg. There are podcasts designed to inspire drowsiness, apps to track your sleep patterns or supply a relaxing soundscape. There are plenty of books to help fix broken sleep and, given that sleep is one of the pillars of good health, you might want to look into all that when you have the energy available.

However, there is another something else — a missing piece of the menopause jigsaw, one that we've known about for a while but quite possibly overlooked — the calming hormone. Progesterone . . .

'People wanting to be 35 when they're 50 makes me think:
Why? Why don't you be 50 and be good at that? And also
embody the kind of choices that are sustainable at that
age.'

— *Emma Thompson*, The Guardian

Chapter 7

It's also about progesterone

For a long time oestrogen was queen, even though we've known about its sister hormone progesterone since early last century.

Progesterone is important for fertility. It's produced by a mass of cells called the corpus luteum, and its job is to make the womb a friendly place for the fertilised egg and ensure that the ovaries don't release any more eggs while a growing foetus is in residence. If you don't get pregnant during that particular menstrual cycle, then the corpus luteum shrinks and levels of progesterone fall, destabilising the lining of the womb and resulting in a menstrual bleed.

Even though oestrogen and progesterone work together all through the fertile years, in menopause treatments oestrogen has dominated. In mainstream medicine, progesterone's usefulness in midlife hormone therapy has been only as a womb protector — it is given as part of HRT to reduce the risks of endometrial cancer that taking supplementary oestrogen brings. And it's the oestrogen that smashes hot flushes and makes everything feel better; that's been the thinking, anyway.

There are signs that this view is changing, and increasingly progesterone is being valued as a useful therapy for women in midlife — so long as it is the right progesterone delivered by the correct route.

The natural health industry got there first. For a while, half the women I knew seemed to be smearing progesterone cream on themselves; they'd been prescribed it by holistic practitioners to relieve everything from mood swings to bloating. Many endocrinologists are pretty dark on this. They say that these creams are produced by compounding pharmacies, which don't have the same controls on them as the pharmaceutical industry, so the dosage — and even the contents — aren't reliable. Also, they say that progesterone isn't absorbed well enough through the skin to be effective when taken that way.

There has always been tension between conventional and alternative medicine, and it seems like progesterone has got caught up in that. But now there is emerging science to suggest that this hormone can be more useful for things like sleep, mood swings, palpitations and even hot flushes than was previously thought.

~

Science can be annoying. It seems like it's always flip-flopping about. One minute something is good for you, the next it isn't. When breakthroughs *do* come, they seem to take forever to actually reach us. But that's just the way science works. There are theories, they get tested, there's a discussion, and then there have to be several more studies that come to the same conclusion, followed by more discussions, before the thinking starts to change. If you're trying to decide what to put into your body right now, of course, none of this is remotely helpful.

The other issue is that scientific studies are written, for the most part, in the most dense and inaccessible way possible. It's almost as if the researchers want to keep the whole thing a big secret. When you actually get to speak to them, most people who have undertaken ground-breaking research are brilliant communicators and very excited about telling the world about their discoveries. But for some reason, academia demands that they write about their findings in a way only other scientists can properly understand. So annoying! And given that we're paying for a lot of that research via charitable donations and tax dollars, also quite rude.

What I can tell you — in plain English — is that experimental studies are suggesting progesterone has potential beyond treating menopause symptoms. It may help brain recovery after a stroke or head injury. And there are experts who believe that it also has scope to treat Parkinson's, multiple sclerosis and Alzheimer's disease. More studies are needed (as researchers are constantly concluding), so this is all for the future.

Thankfully, with menopause the shift is already beginning. Canadian endocrinologist Jerilynn Prior is in the forefront of this. She is the founder of the Centre for Menstrual Cycle and Ovulation Research (CeMCOR), and her work has shown that peri-menopausal symptoms such as sore breasts, weight gain, bloating, heavy periods, migraines, anxiety, sleeplessness, hot flushes, etc., are the result of oestrogen roller-coastering up and down while progesterone is going into a more straightforward decline, putting everything out of balance. She says that body-identical progesterone is safe and effective for women who need help managing these symptoms.

~

As I said earlier, it has to be the right sort of progesterone. The synthetic version — known as progestogen — isn't molecularly identical to the hormone that is produced by our corpus luteum. And Jerilynn Prior isn't advocating that we smear on natural progesterone cream, as in her experience it's not strong enough (or we don't absorb it well enough) to counterbalance the effects of higher oestrogen — so it doesn't seem to do much to reduce hot flushes or improve sleep, and it certainly won't protect the womb if you're taking oestrogen.

The latest advice is that the safest and best version of this hormone to take is a micronised oral progesterone that is body-identical and delivered in oil (sunflower oil in New Zealand). The good news is that a brand called Utrogestan is approved for use here; the less-good news is that it's not subsidised as a menopause treatment. Endocrinologists are lobbying for that to change and very hopeful of success in the near future. In the meantime, oral micronised progesterone is reasonably affordable and worth paying for as part of menopause therapy.

When I say 'reasonably affordable', I'm very aware that some people are on tight budgets and being told that something is only going to cost the equivalent of a few coffees a month may cause them actual pain because café coffees are a luxury. But there is also a lot of cash being splashed around on supplements that have unproven benefits. So while Utrogestan *should* be fully funded, and the independent not-for-profit Best Practice Advocacy Centre New Zealand (bpac[nz]) confirms that it is the better option — and it pisses me off that women are being offered second-best, and I really hope that by the time you read this that has changed — I think we've just got to suck it up and pay for now, if we are able to.

The thing about micronised progesterone is that it needs

to be taken at bedtime because it has a tranquilising effect and makes you very DROWSY. Yes, it will improve sleep. In fact, Jerilynn advises very skinny, sleep-deprived women to begin taking it when they know they can have a lie-in the next day because they might get so much REM sleep that they feel like they have a hangover.

In the brain, micronised progesterone is converted into a metabolite called allopregnanolone, which decreases anxiety and induces sleep. A study led by German researcher Petra Schüssler showed that it helped prevent sleep disturbances in healthy post-menopausal women — participants in this trial had less intermittent wakefulness.[1] (Excuse me while I just roll in the stuff.)

So oestrogen isn't queen after all. In fact, Jerilynn Prior's research has found evidence that using progesterone can be beneficial for many women.[2] As well as leading to more sleep, it can ease hot flushes and night sweats, and reduce menstrual flooding. It doesn't bring an extra risk of clotting, endometrial cancer or depression. Jerilynn believes that a woman can safely take oral micronised progesterone for as long as she needs to, and it may be the only therapy necessary if she is menopausal at a normal age and without risk of osteoporosis.

This isn't a view that I found was shared by New Zealand health medics, probably because 'more research is needed'. GPs and endocrinologists here continue to prescribe progesterone purely as a womb protectant.

The thinking here among mainstream practitioners continues to be that oestrogen can do all the heavy lifting in menopause therapy and progesterone can take it easy. So if you've had a hysterectomy and you go on HRT, you'll be told that you don't need Utrogestan as you have no womb to protect.

The progesterone-only approach is more likely to be taken by integrative health practitioners, who very often offer the hormone in the form of that troublesome cream. I've spoken to loads of women who are convinced that progesterone cream has provided benefits, particularly with sleep, mood and bloating. Possibly they were enjoying a potent placebo effect and the medical argument would be that it's only temporary. But the menopause transition is temporary, too — so if something is safe and is helping get you through, bring it on, right?

The caveat is that the endocrinologists do have a point: with compounded creams, the dosage is unreliable. One doctor told me she had a patient who was getting extraordinarily good results for her hot flushes. Suspicious, the medic sent off a sample of the cream for testing and it turned out to contain oestrogen as well as progesterone. That particular patient had an oestrogen-receptor-positive breast cancer and so using the adulterated cream was dangerous for her.

The progesterone story isn't complete yet. Jerilynn Prior is busy doing more work, as are other researchers.

Potentially, mainstream medicine will follow the natural health industry and start advising progesterone-only therapy during that stage of the menopause transition when oestrogen levels are rising and falling erratically while progesterone has dropped, creating an imbalance. It makes logical sense, but it will take more evidence that it is effective and low-risk before this becomes the accepted and widespread approach.

In the meantime, if you're having heavy flooding or painful periods during peri-menopause you might be offered a hormonal IUD — the Mirena or Jaydess — that contains the synthetic progestogen levonorgestrel, which is a good, safe option.

If you choose to take HRT, you'll be offered progesterone along with the oestrogen only if you still have a womb, to protect against endometrial cancer. However, even if you're post-hysterectomy, it seems like Jerilynn Prior has already provided enough evidence that it may help to take oral micronised progesterone, too, particularly if sleep is a problem. I'd suggest reading more about her work and deciding for yourself. To me it makes logical sense that if the two hormones work in partnership during the fertile years, you'd want to retain the same balance later on.

~

The question is, do you want to take HRT at all? That ought to be an easy one to answer. If you're being tortured by menopause symptoms, you take it; if you're breezing through, then you don't bother. But things are never that black and white — there are always grey areas, and with anything to do with menopause, all that grey seems to have formed a thick bank of fog that can make deciding on the right route to take ridiculously difficult.

Q&A with Canadian endocrinologist Jerilynn Prior

What are we missing here in New Zealand if we're using progesterone in menopause treatment only as a womb protector?

The idea that progesterone might help with menopausal symptom treatment (usually meaning night sweats/hot flushes, called vasomotor symptoms or VMS) but is useful *only* in women with intact wombs is, frankly, bizarre! There are several things that those treating menopausal women need to know:

— When oestrogen therapy for VMS is stopped, at least a quarter of those menopausal women have such a severe withdrawal rebound increase in VMS that they have to re-start oestrogen therapy.[3, 4]

— Progesterone causes no rebound increase in VMS when it is stopped.[5]

— Oestrogen with progesterone/progestin is significantly more effective at controlling VMS than oestrogen alone.[6]

— In women whose uterus and ovaries have been surgically removed (for non-cancer reasons), a randomised, double-blind comparative one-year trial showed that oestrogen and medroxyprogesterone acetate (a progestin) are equally effective at controlling VMS.[7]

Why are we missing this?
Oestrogen was discovered before progesterone. By the time progesterone was discovered, oestrogen was already being used to treat various problems for women and was considered 'the female hormone' to match testosterone as 'the male hormone'. Also, progesterone was not effective when taken by mouth, at least in the doses that were first tried (probably because they didn't realise how much more progesterone than oestrogen is made in the second half of the menstrual cycle).

There were also historically many financial benefits

from oestrogen therapy. In fact, the oestrogen-making companies played an important role in the creation of departments of gynaecology in universities, at least in the United States. So, gynaecologists consider oestrogen to be fundamental and tend to add progesterone only when they are forced to.

Gynaecologists have taught women in general a wrong idea about menstrual cycle hormones — the theme is 'Oestrogen is what makes a girl a girl'. The *right* idea is that oestrogen and progesterone should have balanced actions during the pre-menopausal years.[8] This causes the most regular and least symptomatic menstrual cycles and plays a huge role in optimal fertility. What is also new is that women with the best-balanced oestrogen and progesterone during their menstruating years are least likely to get osteoporosis and fractures, heart attacks and breast and endometrial cancer as they grow older.[8]

What can New Zealand women do?
The only way to overcome misinformation is to replace it with accurate knowledge.

No longer allow doctors to believe that they are the only ones with accurate knowledge. Each woman knows a lot about her own health, especially if she tracks her own experiences. [You can find downloadable menopause and peri-menopause diaries on Jerilynn's website, at www.cemcor. ca/type/diary.] Each woman needs to have done her own research. Then she needs to ask for — and, in fact, *insist on getting* — what she needs. She can frame it this way: 'I'd like to do a trial of progesterone. I've been tracking my hot flushes for such and such a time. If I were to start 300 mg of oral micronised progesterone at bedtime, I can continue to track them and see whether or not they improve. I'll be happy to show you my diary results after three months.'

~

Robyn Malcolm

'Fertility defines so many women.'

Actor Robyn Malcolm has always been a straight-talker, so was unlikely to pass through menopause quietly and invisibly. If she's having a hot flush, she won't act like it's not happening. She's open about her menopause transition being a rough ride at times, and not shy of admitting that for a while there she struggled to cope. Her joints ached, she gained weight, she got hot; but what was happening inside her head was the hardest part.

'I was pretty crippled by it for eighteen months,' she says. 'My whole world shifted. I was psycho with massive mood swings, crying and anxious. And my memory went — I started to panic, thinking I had dementia.'

As a single working mum, Robyn had to keep going, so did whatever she could to help herself during the roughest patch.

'I took bio-identical hormones, which got me through that awful peak,' she says. 'I don't know if it's connected, but I was a very, very happy pregnant person — I think my body likes a lot of hormones. I took magnesium, St John's wort, and did yoga and meditation. And I also took some anti-depressants for a bit.'

Robyn was among the women who said that the end of menstruation took some coming to terms with. Her fertility was a big part of something she had taken for granted: her currency as a woman.

'Fertility defines so many women — *I'm able to have babies, therefore I'm desirable, I'm fit and strong,*' she says. 'When that shifts, it's challenging. I know a lot of people will think it's great when you don't have your period, but I grieved it. I was like:

this is that moment when suddenly I can't have any more children. I used to be able to choose, now I can't.'

Now in her mid-fifties, Robyn is busy raising teenage boys, acting in dramas and launching her own underwear brand (Robyn's Undies), plus she's in love and happy. Right now she feels more secure in herself than ever before. However, she's not interested in pretending that she's living her best life every single moment, even with the worst of the menopause behind her.

'When you've passed through that ring of fire there's an amazing liberation,' she says. 'I hear a lot of women saying it's the greatest time of their life; they're reborn, re-invented. That's true, but it's also one of the biggest challenges that a woman faces. So whenever I have conversations about menopause, I want them to be whole. Yes there's some incredible stuff — but too much "launch into your fifties, you're in your power, it's amazing" risks making those women who are struggling feel like they're failing.'

Is it peri-menopause?
At least 31 symptoms

The signs of 'the change' are wide-ranging, a sort of head-to-toe of biological possibilities. While you may experience some of these symptoms, the good news is you definitely won't have all of them, at least not at the same time.

You may want to add more symptoms of your own at the end of this list. No one really knows how many there are. (One UK endocrinologist, Dr Annice Mukherjee, has suggested that we stop counting, because it's infinite.)

- irregular periods and worsening PMS
- hot flushes
- night sweats
- allergies worsen, or new ones appear
- increased feelings of anxiety or stress
- bloating
- breast tenderness
- brittle nails
- body odour changes
- burning tongue/mouth
- depression

Don't Sweat it

- brain fog
- electric shock sensations under the skin, or brain zaps
- more facial hair; thinning hair on your head
- headaches and migraines
- bladder-control problems
- heart palpitations
- mood swings — rage or tearfulness
- itchy skin
- joint aches and pains
- loss of libido
- loss of confidence
- insomnia
- tingling/pins and needles in extremities
- fatigue
- increase in digestive problems and/or flatulence
- vaginal dryness
- restless leg syndrome
- dizziness
- gum issues — recession, gingivitis, bleeding
- more urinary tract infections

Chapter 8

Why is it all so hard? (A short history of HRT)

If you've got a headache you take paracetamol, if your knees are stuffed you take an anti-inflammatory drug, if you've got high cholesterol you take a statin, if you don't want to get pregnant you use some form of contraception. If you have debilitating menopause symptoms, it's not that simple. It should be. But it isn't.

It's not as if menopause comes out of nowhere as a big surprise. It's there, waiting on the horizon, and if we're biologically female and make it to midlife, then we'll crash into it eventually.

Menopause has had a long history of being misunderstood. If you think it's tricky getting the right treatment now, spare a thought for some of our eighteenth-century sisters who were subject to the most heinous cures. The male physicians of the time thought that the lack of periods — known as courses back then — was because the blood had somehow got stuck up there and so needed to be purged to prevent it stagnating. Leeches were attached to the genitalia and cervix to help this along. *Leeches!* Women were blistered, cut and cauterised. They were advised to eat 'cooling' diets and avoid inappropriate excitement. Some were told not to have sex. Or take tepid baths. Injections of ice water into the rectum or ice applied to the vagina were used to calm a condition that was believed could cause insanity, hysteria, mania, melancholia, apathy, and more! Some doctors even experimented with ovarian extracts taken from pigs or cows, but not with any degree of knowing what they were doing. No wonder this became a time of life for women to dread.

Generally it was only wealthy women who could afford to visit physicians for these hideous treatments, so this was one of the few situations where it seemed an advantage to be poor. Cash-strapped women just got on with it, which was without doubt the better option at the time.

These days, though, women don't have to 'just get on with it'. Last century, medical researchers got to grips with hormones and how they work — and the idea of replacing them, once they went missing, really took hold.

HRT was a huge success story for a while. By the 1990s a huge number of women were on it. Possibly the reason our mothers' generation never bothered talking about 'the change' is because they were so hormonally boosted that they weren't having problems. HRT was considered to be a safe and efficient way to deal to hot flushes and also to protect against the health problems of later life, like the brittle-bone disease osteoporosis, cardiovascular disease and even dementia. Hormones made you look and feel younger, your husband would like you more and you'd be crazy not to take them — that seemed to be the prevailing attitude.

The game-changer was a study called the Woman's Health Initiative (WHI).[1] A lot has been written about this study and you can easily do a deep-dive if you like, so consider this as a fairly brisk briefing.

First of all, it's important to know that the hormone replacement therapy arm of the WHI study wasn't about proving that it helped with symptoms like hot flushes: women had already made it abundantly clear that it did. What the researchers were interested in discovering was whether it also provided protection against heart disease and the fractured brittle bones of osteoporosis. Also, obviously, they were monitoring for any risks.

There had already been a smaller trial that suggested

there were benefits to heart health, and now researchers were looking to see if they got the same result with a larger group of people — which is how science works. The WHI was a randomised, placebo-controlled trial with 161,000 women participating and was funded by the US government, not a pharmaceutical company, so this was gold-standard science.

In 2002, five years into the study, it was halted amid a blaze of publicity because it seemed there had actually been an *increase* in heart attacks and strokes among the group of women taking HRT. The real kicker, though, was that according to the WHI study, the women on HRT had a 24% greater risk of invasive breast cancer than those getting the placebo over six to seven years. That was what hit the headlines and changed everyone's thinking.

Even at the time, though, there was controversy. I listened to a really interesting podcast (well, interesting once the preliminary whiffle was over — why do podcasters have to do that?) with Professor Robert Langer who was involved with the WHI trial, and it takes us behind the scenes to look at what happened.[2] He says that not all of the researchers agreed with the paper that was published or the press release that was sent out. They tried to get both changed, but it was too late.

People freaked out. Women flushed their hormone supplements down the toilet, lawsuits starting flying around; basically it was one big drama and HRT's reputation was shot. The mantra from then on became 'the lowest dose for the shortest period', and a lot of doctors were very nervous about prescribing HRT at all.

As a result, there is no doubt that some women have suffered unnecessarily. Because what we now know is that the picture is bigger. When people started drilling down into the research, they discovered that *when* you start taking HRT is an important factor.

The WHI participants were aged between 50 and 79. A lot of them were much older than is typical for women taking hormone therapy to alleviate menopause symptoms. They were post-menopausal; some a long way past menopause. Most crucially, only 33% of them were under 60. It turned out that these younger women, in the age band where you'd be most likely to need HRT, actually had a reduced risk of heart disease. And their extra breast cancer risk was not especially significant.

Hormones aren't a miracle youth-restorer. And it seems that if a woman has been without them for a long time, then there is more harm than good in re-introducing them to her body. For a younger woman, starting the therapy closer to menopause, there are fewer risks and more benefits. This 'window of safety' is now a part of the updated guidelines.

If you are below 60 or within ten years of your last menstrual period, with no other major risk factors, then HRT is considered fine for your heart and an appropriate treatment for your hot flushes/night sweats. There are other benefits, too. HRT helps prevent osteoporosis, lowers the risk of bowel cancer and type 2 diabetes, keeps the vagina perky (remember GSM?) and, while the jury is still very much out on dementia, it may help brain health. It also improves sleep and mood. Possibly that might be a domino effect from reducing the flushes, etc. But if you're more rested and less enraged/weepy/depressed, then you're probably not tying yourself in knots wondering about the exact mechanism.

And now back to the WHI. The other issue with the study is that the women involved were taking an older form of HRT, an oral oestrogen derived from the purified urine of pregnant mares, called Premarin, and a synthetic progestogen called Provera.

Those who care about animal welfare won't want a bar of an oestrogen product that animal-rights organisation PETA says is produced by impregnating hundreds of thousands of horses, then standing them in a stall with sacks strapped to their groins and restricting their water intake so that their urine becomes concentrated. The foals they have eleven months after conceiving are considered a by-product and are mostly slaughtered for horse meat or dog food. Fortunately, there are modern plant-based forms of hormones available, and Christchurch endocrinologist Anna Fenton told me she hasn't prescribed Premarin for twenty years. When I say plant-based, let's be clear that these are still very synthetic products — we're not talking green smoothies here. These hormones are made in a lab out of stuff extracted from wild yam, flax and soy. But they are still an improvement on the hormones used in the WHI study.

Also, oestrogen patches don't carry the same clotting/ stroke risk as oestrogen taken orally as a pill. And the molecularly identical form of micronised progesterone, brand name Utrogestan, is believed to have less breast cancer risk than the old-style progestogens.

'They are exactly the same as the hormones the body would have produced prior to menopause,' says Anna. 'You're giving back what is missing, not a poor copy of it.'

The oestrogen patch funded and most commonly prescribed in New Zealand is called Estradot. It comes in various doses and can be cut into different sizes if you want to tailor the dose to a woman's specific needs.

~

Even though the treatment has evolved in the twenty years since the WHI study, the breast cancer risk with HRT hasn't disappeared entirely. For many women it is a very small risk, but still it needs to be considered. Hormone therapy can also thicken the breast tissue, which makes mammograms less accurate.

To add to the confusion, in 2019 a study was published in medical journal *The Lancet* that raised the breast cancer issue again.[3] It came from a group of UK epidemiologists called the Collaborative Group on Hormonal Factors in Menopause, and pooled data from a number of different studies, including the WHI. The final line states: 'In western countries there have been about 20 million breast cancers diagnosed since 1990, of which about 1 million would have been caused by MHT [menopausal hormone therapy] use.'

Frankly, that is enough to put anyone off. But experts ripped into the study, saying that most of it was based on the older forms of hormones, that some of the studies were observational and that other factors might have been responsible. The Australasian Menopause Society's position on this particular piece of research was that the breast cancer risks had been exaggerated.

Oestrogen therapy alone doesn't appear to be linked to an elevated risk of breast cancer. It is when progestogens are added that the problem arises. And if you have a womb, then you need progestogens as a protectant (it prevents the lining of the womb becoming too thick, which raises the risk of endometrial cancer). It sounds like a Catch-22 situation, except that there does seem to be a lower risk for women who take progesterone cyclically — i.e. more closely mimicking the way it would be naturally released in the body. And the other issue is that most of the women reviewed in the research were taking the old synthetic progestogens, not the safer body-identical micronised progesterone which studies so far have suggested has no increased risk.[4] Guess what? More research is needed.

This is what the Australasian Menopause Society says about hormone therapy and breast cancer risk at the time of writing this book (2021), although obviously things are always subject to change.[5]

- Different progestogens have different risk ratios for breast cancer. Micronised progesterone appears safer than most synthetic progestogens.
- In women prescribed HRT close to the menopause and for short-term use (up to five years), there were three extra cases per 10,000 women-years for oestrogen alone and nine extra cases per 10,000 women-years for oestrogen plus progestogen. The risk is increased with longer duration of use, particularly in older women (over age 60). The risk decreased after HRT was ceased.
- Obesity increases the risk of breast cancer. HRT use in obese women does not further increase their risk.
- Recent studies have demonstrated no increased risk of breast cancer with vaginal oestrogen.

Breast cancer is one of those highly emotive conditions. A lot of women die of things like heart disease and osteoporosis, but bones and cardiac muscles aren't sexy, they don't suckle babies, and saving your life doesn't involve surgically removing them.

All of us know women who have had breast cancer. One of my best friends died in her early forties, and since then lots of other women who I care about have been through treatment. Interestingly, as far as I know, none of them was on HRT. But in the course of researching this book I did come across a few women who developed breast cancer after taking hormones. The two things might not have been related, but these women couldn't help worrying that they were and, to some degree, blaming themselves.

There are a lot of statistics flying about, depending on which form of HRT you're on and how long you take it for, but you are not a statistic and your risk is not going to be exactly the same as that for the woman sitting next to you.

We also need to think about the other risks our everyday lives are exposing us to (whether or not we plan to take HRT).

Alcohol is linked with several cancers, including breast cancer,[6] but how many of us take that into account when we pop a bottle of bubbles and clink glasses? It contains acetaldehyde, a probable human carcinogen that is also in a lot of other things, including food preservatives and flavourings according to our Environmental Protection Agency (EPA). As mentioned earlier, alcohol also keeps our ageing, shrinking livers busy, and as they focus on eliminating the introduced toxin they neglect other jobs such as breaking down oestrogen. That means higher levels of hormone are free to float around in our bodies and potentially affect our tissues.

In 2017 the American Institute for Cancer Research (AICR) and the World Cancer Research Fund (WCRF) released a report that said just one alcoholic drink a day increases breast cancer risk by 5% in pre-menopausal women and 9% in post-menopausal ones.[7] They also found that being obese increased the risk, as does being inactive. The good news is that exercise lowered the risk by 17% for pre-menopausal women and 10% for post menopausal women. Breastfeeding also helps reduce a woman's chance of breast cancer, and there is some evidence that a diet rich in non-starchy vegetables and carotonoids — carrots, apricots, spinach, kale — has a protective effect.

There are many things outside of our control, of course. Daily we're exposed to different combinations of endocrine-disrupting chemicals and no one fully understands what risks they bring. And, of course, some women have a strong family history of breast cancer and carry genes that make them more likely to develop it, so hormone therapies are not advised for them at all.

Weighing up risks and benefits is a part of any medical treatment you choose to take. Aspirin prevents blood clots so lowers the risk of heart attack and stroke, but it also erodes the stomach lining and increases the chance of a bleed in the brain. Paracetamol blocks pain signals to the brain, and since you can buy it easily at a supermarket most of us have some around the house — which is probably why it's one of the most common substances involved in childhood poisoning. There is a risk with anything you take, and you are the only one who has the right to decide whether the benefits outweigh that risk. Or not.

In life there are always people trying to tell you what to do, and with menopause that is supercharged. One opinion you may come across is that menopause is a natural part of life so you shouldn't medicalise it (the people saying that probably aren't the ones waking throughout the night soaked in sweat and shivering). Then there is the idea that taking HRT is like bathing in a fountain of youth, so you must only want it if you're vain and care too much about having nice skin. You'll come across well-meaning people with an alternative therapy that has worked for them, so they insist that you absolutely definitely must try it. You'll find misinformation and scare stories, and be targeted by businesses, large and small, that want to make money out of you and your menopause symptoms.

Why is it all so hard? (A short history of HRT)

~

Why is it all so hard? Well, all of the above are some of the reasons. Then there are the challenges of actually getting treated. The hangover from the WHI study is still raging out there. A lot of doctors who are practising now will have trained during the years when HRT was considered a huge no-no, and they remain very wary of it. You've got to have some sympathy: these are busy people and the updated position statements of international menopause societies aren't exactly bedtime reading. Many of them haven't had anywhere near enough training in this area. And in the information aimed at them there are conflicting facts and inconsistent advice.

Doctors don't want to do harm, so I can sympathise with those who are shy of hormone therapy. But if it means that women are struggling to get the care they need, then there needs to be a change.

'There is only one GP in my practice who prescribes HRT, and there's a long wait for an appointment,' one woman told me.

'It's three months before I can see an endocrinologist,' said another.

'My doctor told me that Utrogestan was only available for pregnant women to prevent miscarriage.'

'I wanted HRT, but my doctor would only give me an anti-depressant.'

That was the sort of thing I was hearing, so I asked around to see if it was an accurate picture of the landscape out there. 'Yes!' came the reply.

There are people trying to do something about it. South Auckland GP Orna McGinn has a strong interest in women's health, and along with the Gender Justice Collective she has been calling for a National Women's Health Strategy to create a system that is easier for women to navigate, not just in menopause but throughout our fertile years.

'I think the access for women to really, really good menopause care is limited,' she says. 'There are lots of reasons for that. There is not a lot of good training for GPs around menopause, which is amazing when you think that every single one of their female patients is going to go through it. But all of women's health is lacking. It's a real black hole, unfortunately. Prescribing HRT is very straightforward, so it's a shame if women are being turned away.'

They've even changed its name now. We're meant to call it MHT, meaning menopausal hormone therapy. That smells like a rebrand, but the official line is that it's more accurate on the grounds that you're not restoring hormones to the same level they were at during your fertile years, only putting enough back in to ease the transition. Whatever. Prince tried changing his name to a symbol and that didn't take either. Once you're famous as something, you're famous. Doctors may call it MHT, but almost everyone else is sticking with the old name.

Women have a right to be pissed off if there is a widely available therapy that has been proven to be safe for many but they are having difficulties getting it. That certainly seems to be the case for many in Aotearoa presently — the pendulum is still stuck in the position it swung to after the WHI study scared everyone.

In other places the HRT pendulum seems to be swinging back again dramatically. In the UK there is a specialist called Louise Newson who runs a private menopause and wellness clinic staffed by a team that includes a pelvic floor physiotherapist, a yoga teacher and a nutritionist, as well as doctors and nurses. She is making a lot of noise about the challenges of menopause — apparently, during her own transition she was so irritable that she couldn't even stand the sound of her husband breathing — and she's launched a free app called balance, as well as the website My Menopause Doctor, both brimming with information. Louise Newson is very much pro-HRT (verging on evangelical), talking and writing constantly about its benefits. I listened to one podcast where she spoke of prescribing hormones to women who are in their sixties, seventies, even one in her nineties. I've also heard her and other experts describe menopause as a 'long-term hormone deficiency'. Hmmm. That word 'deficiency' implies that there is something wrong with us, a condition that requires medicalising to save us — not that we are experiencing a very natural part of the ageing process. It sounds too much like a sales pitch to me. And I'm starting to feel a little concerned.

While it's definitely time to redress the balance, there is a danger that the pendulum might swing too far and we'll go back to the idea that HRT is the best and only therapy for all midlife women, and you might as well put it in the water supply. I'm not sure if that's much better than the current habit of over-stating the risks and minimising the benefits.

A wildly swinging pendulum is no help to anyone. Science evolves; we all get that. The menopause story is still developing, and in the future things might shift again. But right at this moment, if we're already dealing with wildly fluctuating hormones then we need some clear messaging to help us make a decision that's right for us, right now.

Q&A with Auckland endocrinologist Stella Milsom

So is HRT back on the table?

Yes, I think it is. For a symptomatic woman who is under the age of 60, within ten years of menopause, and whose quality of life is being affected, you should be discussing hormone replacement unless there is a good reason not to, which would be either because the woman didn't want to use it or because of one of the very few contraindications to hormone use.

What are the medical reasons not to use HRT?
Previous breast cancer, undiagnosed vaginal bleeding, active liver disease, a high-grade cancer of the womb that might be oestrogen-sensitive, and potentially a prior history of a blood clot, stroke or heart attack. All of which, in the age group that are symptomatic, by and large are going to be pretty unusual.

How common is it for women's menopause symptoms to be bad enough to need medical help?
The rule of thumb is that a quarter of women will pass through menopause without really noticing, a quarter of women are going to have really miserable symptoms that seriously affect their quality of life and their functioning, and the other 50% are going to be somewhere in between — so that's a lot of women who potentially might need at least a discussion about alleviating their symptoms.

The peri-menopausal woman, who is earlier in the transition, may have a slightly different set of symptoms that seem more like PMT, so breast tenderness, bloating, moodiness, the skin crawling — the clue is that the periods have started to become erratic. And then you might have a woman who's just in bits, can't understand how she's gone from a highly functioning professional to not being able to sleep, getting flushes, brain fog. These cognitive symptoms are very common, actually, such as lower mood, new onset of anxiety, but also things like brain fog, losing the ability to put names to people, not able to read a spreadsheet that you could normally do — and it causes a lot of distress. Also musculoskeletal symptoms [aches and pains] are not uncommon and often aren't attributed to menopause.

In your experience, are a lot of women still struggling to get the right treatment?
Well, I'm not seeing the happy patients who have already been prescribed hormones! Every day or week a new referral comes in. Last week I saw a woman who was told she couldn't have MHT because her periods hadn't stopped; the week before, someone who had been told she couldn't have hormones because of migraines. Women are told that these symptoms are part of natural ageing and it will all disappear, or told to have a holiday or go on anti-depressants. It is distressing

to see the misery and frustration of women who have been to several different practitioners and hormones haven't been mentioned once, even though they might be an ideal candidate.

There is the breast cancer risk, though?
It's a very small additional risk and you have to balance it out with some significant positives. If you're a menopausal woman who's otherwise healthy and you're having a wretched time, I think the data remains very clear on the balance of benefits to that woman. It makes a huge difference if a woman can sleep, that her mood improves, her anxiety disappears, her flushes go away. I think we really do under-estimate how miserable these symptoms are and how much symptoms influence quality of life.

You've also got potential benefits on other health issues. Osteoporosis prevention, bowel cancer prevention, diabetes prevention, probably cardiac prevention, particularly if a woman is taking oestrogen alone. So I think we've got quite a lot of positives. Also you can potentially mitigate the breast cancer risk by altering the route by which you take the hormones [oestrogen patches rather than pills], using natural progesterone, having regular mammogram screening, and living a healthier lifestyle. Being sedentary, overweight and drinking moderate amounts of alcohol all increase breast cancer risk at least as much as hormones do.

When should you stop taking the hormones?

There's no rule that says you must stop after five years or by the time you're 60. Around 40% of women will continue to flush. If a woman is healthy, she's a better candidate than one who has put on a lot of weight and developed metabolic syndrome [obesity, high blood pressure, high cholesterol, high blood sugar]. I'm increasingly finding it hard to justify discontinuing hormone use in my patients who have been on it for some years and want to continue. We know that after eighteen years of hormone use there is no excess mortality from hormones, whether from breast cancer or anything else [because studies showing more breast cancer don't show more women dying from it], which is very encouraging data.

Peta Mathias

'I don't believe in suffering if you don't have to.'

Peta Mathias is completely fabulous. In her early seventies, she is a writer, a cook, an adventurer, a performer and one of those women who lives stylishly no matter what. Peta isn't the slightest bit interested in conforming to other people's ideas of who she should be and how she should behave, and when it came to midlife she very determinedly chose her own path.

'When I was 50 I went to my doctor and said I don't want to have another period in my life so put me on a dosage of HRT that stops them,' explains Peta. 'Over time that dosage has been changed but it's suited me, I've had no bad effects yet. I don't believe in suffering if you don't have to, so I'm still taking it because every time I try to stop I get terrible hot flushes and wild night sweats. I'm tired of putting pills in my mouth and patches on my belly, so I've slowly, slowly decreased the dose — but, of course, it gets to the point where your body realises you're trying to trick it and you get the flushes again.'

A downside of midlife for Peta was that her weight crept up. 'I gained more than a kilo a year in menopause,' she says. 'My normal weight is 60 kilos and I went up to 75. Maybe it was a combination of not being in menopause anymore and travelling a lot in India where it was too hot to eat, but that seemed to break the problem. The really cruel thing is we don't need to eat as much as we age.'

These days Peta is fitting into clothes she couldn't wear for years (and she has some amazing clothes). She enjoys food, but skips breakfast and serves smaller portions. And although she hates exercise, she forces herself to do it and feels great afterwards.

Reaching midlife wasn't too much of a mental adjustment, says Peta, as she had her midlife crisis early. 'I like to think I'm ahead of the crowd! When I was about 30 I had this moment when I looked in the mirror and thought, "What are you doing? Your body is changing, your hair is losing its colour . . . have you done enough? Get your act together, make some changes."'

And so Peta created the life she still leads today, writing books and leading gastronomic tours around the world (or around Aotearoa during the pandemic with overseas travel not possible), performing a one-woman show and teaching cooking classes. There are no plans to retire because she likes to feel as though she is contributing to the world. Neither is Peta likely to stop having adventures and tackling new challenges.

'I still feel that I haven't reached my peak yet and I've got lots of interesting things I have to do yet with my life,' she says. 'I think that attitude helps you through menopause and midlife.'

'I always thought menopause was going to be the end of the earth. But it is so not — it's the opposite. You have this incredible energy, and you can still feel sexy and fabulous . . . but there is a freedom that comes with it.'

— *Annabel Langbein,* The Australian Women's Weekly

Chapter 9

To HRT or not to HRT? That is the question

The middle-aged female body requires so much maintenance it's exhausting. I wish I could just go to one place and get the whole lot done – mammogram, smear test, teeth checked, grey roots retouched, maybe a bit of Botox, definitely a restorative facial, and since my toenails now seem to be too far from my head, could someone please take a look down there and find out what needs doing?

I'm never going to get my one-stop shop for midlife healthcare and beauty. Nor am I likely to find a menopause clinic where they also have a yoga teacher — at least not yet. What I have access to is a health system that has served me well in the past when things have gone wrong.

A day after being diagnosed with a broken ankle, I was in surgery. When I had a really nasty corneal ulcer, the hospital care I got was prompt and effective. So I have faith that the help is out there for the menopause transition, if you know where to look and how to ask for it.

Wanting and needing HRT isn't the only reason to take your menopause symptoms to a doctor. For a start, there may something else going on. There are all sorts of reasons for fatigue, for instance, including low iron and underactive thyroid or possibly more serious conditions.

Midlife is an ideal time to check in with your body. Maybe do some blood tests to make sure iron levels are good, check that cholesterol, blood sugar, etc, are all tracking okay. While you're at the doctor get your blood pressure checked; and, in your own time, assess how well you're doing on the self-care front. And if you need help with menopause symptoms, then ask for it.

Doctors aren't satanic slaves of the pharmaceutical industry. They will talk through non-drug options, like hypnosis and CBT, and some are happy to work hand-in-hand with a naturopath and medical herbalist. If you're in distress but you don't want to take hormones, then there are other drugs that might help. What you need is a healthcare provider who listens and is open to all the options.

– The Australasian Menopause Society has a page where it lists New Zealand doctors who are members, but there aren't very many of them, and if we all try to book in at once there's going to be a serious logjam. You'll find a link to the page, along with a list of other useful websites, at the end of the book.

- Your GP is qualified to prescribe HRT, but still might be hesitant. Some would prefer not to touch it at all. If that's the case, and you've made a decision that you want to take hormones but you're not getting them, then change your GP. You want someone who is confident and skilled in this area, not a nervous non-expert. Ideally you'll find a medical professional who will work with a registered medical herbalist or naturopath if you're using one.

- Other women are your best resource at this point. Ask around in your network of friends — someone is bound to have a recommendation. If not, there are increasing numbers of social media groups bristling with midlife women. Menopause Over Martinis is one with a lot of Aotearoa-based members. It has a very active Facebook page as well as holding events like potluck dinners that bring women together.

You may not feel 100% comfortable bringing up the subject of menopause with friends and family members. I, on the other hand, am heroically forthright. Since embarking on the research for this book I have asked pretty much every middle-aged woman I've come across about her experience. Most seemed keen to share the details. Some were very funny. A couple were in denial about being peri-menopausal (but we've all been there). A few were through the whole thing and had hardly noticed. Some told stories of the sweat flying off their foreheads and spattering passers-by. No one was offended.

If there was a conspiracy of silence about menopause, then it's been well and truly broken. To be honest, I'm not sure if I buy into the whole 'no one talks about it' narrative. That hasn't been entirely true for quite some time. In the early 1990s Gail Sheehy published *The Silent Passage* and Germaine Greer wrote her polemic *The Change. Menopause the Musical* premiered in 2001 — and if people were singing about it, then surely they were talking about it? Possibly the problem was that the rest of us were trying really, really hard not to listen.

There is such a cacophony of noise being made about menopause now — not only by social media groups, but also podcasts, TV shows, blogs, websites, email newsletters (hotflashinc.com is great). Even celebrities are talking about it — Salma Hayek says her breasts got bigger during the menopause transition. Michelle Obama revealed that she had a hot flush while travelling on the presidential helicopter. Oprah Winfrey has discussed her midlife insomnia and heart palpitations. Kim Cattrall addressed the fear of no longer being desirable, attractive and feminine. Gwyneth Paltrow has admitted to rage with no reason.

To HRT or not to HRT? That is the question

So I think it's fine to ask a casual acquaintance if she's on hormones and, if so, how it's going and where she got them.

~

The question is, though, do you want to take the hormones? If there are no known health risks and you are among the 25% who are having a horrible time, then the decision may be an easy one. Some women told me they practically crawled on their hands and knees into their doctor's surgery, pleading 'Give me the hormones now.'

Weighing up the pros and cons gets trickier if you're in the 50% of women who are soldiering on but not feeling amazing most of the time. That's when you have to start recording your symptoms and deciding how much they are affecting your day-to-day life. Personally, I like making lists. And so, since I'd put myself in the 50% group, my list right now goes like this:

- Hot flushes — feel like I'm through the worst of it, palpitations aren't as bad, don't get night sweats, not really bothering me and was never unbearable.
- Mood swings — haven't yelled at a random stranger in ages. Suspect all the people who are annoying me now genuinely are very annoying. Am quite anxious but possibly for legitimate reasons.
- Sleep — still a bit shit although melatonin helps, as does limiting caffeine and alcohol intake.

- Fatigue — yes I must get around to going for those blood tests to check my iron levels and thyroid function.
- Bone health — yes I must get around to going for that scan to check my bone density.
- Aches and pains — I did get my sore knees and hips checked, and it turns out I've got osteoarthritis, which isn't very sexy but at least menopause is off the hook for that one.
- Dryness — I'm like a chip: my hair, my skin, I'm practically crispy. Every external part of me is being moisturised to within an inch of its life and I suspect my vagina is next.
- Periods — all done with and I've thrown out the last dusty tampons. In peri-menopause heavy periods did affect my life so I should have done something about it.
- Breast cancer risk — some family history, I'm a bit overweight, and limiting the wine isn't going quite as well as it should.
- General concerns — I had a whopping migraine the last time I took the combined pill, and although that was ages ago, half my body went numb and I thought I was having a stroke, so the memory lingers and puts me off taking more hormones (rightly or wrongly).
- Decision — no HRT for now.

I'm naturally drug-adverse. Blame my mother, who was still offering me junior aspirin for headaches when I was in my thirties. And my father, whose response to most ills is to make you drink freshly squeezed lemon juice or press a leaf to your skin. We just aren't a medication family. However, even a couple of years ago that list of mine wouldn't have been the same.

If every woman is different, then so is every stage of the menopause transition.

I've come across various ways of breaking it down. They may use different language, but they all pretty much say the same thing and it's based on STRAW (Stages of Reproductive Ageing Workshop) — a system devised by a bunch of menopause experts to help identify where we're at.

- Pre-menopause — you're still having regular periods.
- Early peri-menopause — you're noticing changes to your menstrual cycle.
- Late peri-menopause — your cycle is much more irregular. You may start skipping periods, and this is when mood swings, migraines, itchiness, tiredness and the other niggly symptoms tend to start up. It is possible to not recognise the signs until you start getting the hot flushes.
- Early post-menopause — you haven't had a period for twelve months, but you may well still be flushing and having night sweats, sleeplessness, brain fog, etc.

- Late post-menopause — hopefully by now the worst of the flushing, etc, is over, although this is when GSM (genitourinary syndrome of menopause, remember?) puts in an appearance with more chance of vaginal dryness, thinning of the vaginal wall, and more urinary tract infections.

It's said that the menopause transition lasts eight to ten years, but actually this whole process might drag on through decades of a woman's life, although some will be more aware of it than others.

In the early stages, the regularity of your natural menstrual cycle is the best clue. But if you're using a hormonal contraceptive such as the combined pill, the implant (also known as 'the rods') or the Depo-Provera injection, then you won't know what your natural cycle is.

I'm not suggesting that you give up using contraceptives. The advice on this differs, depending where you look, but the Australasian Menopause Society says that women are at risk of an unintended pregnancy until twelve months after their last menstrual period if they're over the age of 50 and for 24 months if they're under 50. It's generally accepted that once you're 55 you can stop (my husband has been strangely reluctant, even though I've assured him that if I did conceive at this stage we could sell our miracle baby story to a woman's magazine and probably score free nappies).

It's also important to know that oestrogen-containing contraceptive methods (like the combined pill and the injection) are generally not recommended after the age of 50, as then the cardiovascular risks outweigh the benefits.

Today many women are only just getting around to starting their families at 35 when it's likely that they are also moving into that first pre-menopausal stage, but there are no hard and fast rules. For some it all happens too soon, which is both emotionally and physically tough. That does make the hormone therapy decision a little more straightforward, though, at least to begin with.

Primary ovarian insufficiency (POI) is the term used when menstrual periods stop before the age of 40. This happens to about 4% of women, and around twelve in every 100 women will have a spontaneous early menopause between the ages of 40 and 45. Often there's no known reason why, although it can be genetic, caused by an infection or autoimmune condition, or related to polycystic ovarian syndrome (PCOS). In some women it is surgically induced (e.g. following an oophorectomy, which is surgery to remove the ovaries).

Obviously, if you're hoping to get pregnant then fertility will be the first thing you consider, but you also need to think about the impact on your body because POI increases your risk of long-term health problems related to cardiovascular disease and osteoporosis. For this reason women who go into early menopause are advised to consider hormone therapy, to replace what has been prematurely lost, and continue until the typical age of menopause — around 52. Whether you continue after that will involve the same risk/benefit analysis every other woman with significant menopause symptoms needs to go through.

Diagnosis of POI can be tricky, as both doctors and women might not consider the possibility of menopause in someone who is young. If you're under 40, you should get checked if you haven't had a period in four months — this will involve testing blood to assess your levels of follicle-stimulating hormone (FSH), and since it's another hormone that fluctuates you'll have more than one test.

~

There are so many bad news stories about hormone therapy, but I talked to a lot of women who were taking it and they were overwhelmingly positive. They didn't find the oestrogen patches difficult or messy to use, and were convinced that they felt better because of it. One woman told me that at first she almost felt like she was high on drugs, although that wore off (this was most likely a reflection of how deeply awful she'd felt before). The oldest woman I found had turned 80. A professional, still working part-time in her chosen career and with a very full life, she had no plans to give up because she believed that the hormones were giving her the energy to continue living the way she wanted to.

I'm absolutely not trying to push HRT — your healthcare choices are up to you. All I care about is your right to make that choice backed with the best information available. But if you *have* decided to give it a go, then you can start on a low dose and remain on it for a short time to get you through the worst patch. You don't have to commit to it forever.

For some of you, it may be that there is a family history of osteoporosis and heart problems, and you are hoping for some protection from longer-term health problems. What you should know, though, is that 'the lowest dose for the shortest time' mantra is still being repeated. Also, most doctors will prescribe hormones to treat severe hot flushes but not any other disease or symptoms.

So if you are set on HRT, don't bother mentioning your interest in the benefit to your bones or your hopes of staving off diabetes or dementia. If you're struggling with mood swings and sleeplessness, it's best not to bring them up either or else you'll be offered other options — like anti-depressants.

In your precious fifteen minutes of GP face-time it pays to stay on message. Have a diary of your flushes, with information about frequency and severity. Make it clear how much this is affecting your life and overall health. Also show an understanding of the risk factors. But mainly talk about being hot, hot, hot. This is the thing most likely to score you the hormones you're asking for, from your pressured, short-on-time and possibly over-cautious GP.

Endocrinologist Stella Milsom told me that she spends an hour with a new menopause patient, which will include giving her information and further reading, and there will be follow-up consultations. You shouldn't need to go and see a specialist endocrinologist. But it may take more than one GP visit to get your dose right, and you may want to review where you're at on a regular basis.

There are other drugs that can be prescribed to treat individual symptoms — see the Q&A with endocrinologist Anna Fenton for more — but no patch or pill is a miracle. Everything that has an effect has the potential for side-effects and nothing makes up for an unhealthy lifestyle.

Don't worry, this isn't where I start preaching. We all know we need to eat healthily and that exercise is good, etc, etc. If that's news to anyone at this point, the rock they have been living under must have been enormous. But in midlife, as your body changes so too does the things it needs. And I think (in a non-preachy and non-bodyshaming way), that it's worth exploring that a bit more.

Q&A with Christchurch endocrinologist Anna Fenton

Are people still rattled about HRT?

Yes, they are. I think the problem is that the media did such a good job of increasing anxiety. Once people have fixed ideas — and that applies to doctors as well as to women — it's very hard to change them back again. Women have been left with the idea that they have no options at all; they just have to grit their teeth and keep going. It's almost become a feminist issue, that you just have to tough it out. But there's such a wide range of options women can take. It's not just that you have to take HRT or nothing at all — there are quite simple complementary or prescription therapies available. So I think it's important to let women know they've got options and if they're having symptoms, don't suffer — look into what those options might be.

So what are some of those other options?

There's a wide variety. There is some pretty good evidence for things like hypnosis. People are often surprised when I bring that up. Cognitive behavioural therapy [CBT] and mindfulness seem to affect not just how women cope with things like flushes but also the severity of the symptoms themselves. There are also some effective complementary or herbal options, particularly for managing mood. This includes maca root and St John's wort. Then you move on to things that we can prescribe as doctors. They are largely drugs that we use off-label as they are licensed for other things, like treating over-active bladders, back pain or depression, but they also help manage menopausal symptoms.

The one we prescribe the most these days would be oxybutynin, which has been around for probably 50 years to treat over-active bladders. It's not very effective at doing that, so it's always been a drug that's looked for a purpose. It works really well for hot flush control and you don't need much of it. Really the only downside is you get a dry mouth, but generally people tolerate it very well and it's very safe, so we use that quite a lot for flushing. Unfortunately, there have been supply issues worldwide [during the Covid-19 pandemic] so it's not easily available.

The SSRI anti-depressant family is quite effective at dealing with mood, flushes and sleep at menopause. For women who have had breast cancer, they can be very useful. As soon as you use the word 'anti-depressant' a lot of people don't want to take them, but they can work really well.

Then there's gabapentin, which has been around for a while to deal with epilepsy and neuropathic pain. We use it a bit to reduce hot flushes, but it can make women feel a bit spaced-out and that can be a problem. It has to be weaned down very slowly, so it would be my last choice in terms of things we can prescribe.

Down here in Christchurch we also do a nerve block. There is a ganglion or bundle of nerves that comes close to the surface at the base of the neck, and you can inject a local anaesthetic into that which reduces hot flushes for many women for months on end. For the post-cancer group who are used to having medical procedures, we do offer that.

If a woman is on HRT, how often would you review it?

Once we've started someone on hormone therapy, I'll say let me know if there's any immediate problem, then update me in three or four weeks. This is because you've generally started with quite low doses, and at that point, once the women are getting a feel for how things are going, you may want to adjust this. I do a lot of that by phone, email and Zoom. Then I'd get them back in after three months so that we can see them physically and check blood pressure, weight and things like that. Once they're stable, either the GP or we can see them at yearly intervals and assess how much longer they need to be on it.

What can you do to help the drop in sex drive?

That's a really big issue, and it's one of those things I ask everybody about because it's not something they're usually going to bring up the first time you meet them. It's a really complicated issue in women. It's not just a hormonal thing. The best evidence we've got is that life probably has more impact on libido in women than hormones do, but that's where menopause makes a difference. If you're tired, if you've gained weight and you don't think you look particularly attractive to your partner, if you're hot and probably a bit grumpy, there are all these things that feed into it — let alone the hormonal changes, the dryness and the discomfort of having sex. It's about trying to pick that apart when you're talking to women. How much is it that you're so dog-tired that you want to go to sleep, how much is it that there's pain and discomfort? And how much is this bothering you or does it bother your partner more — who are you doing it for?

I think getting 'down below' comfortable so that there's no pain and dryness, that's a big part of it. Getting women to sleep so they've got their energy back; that helps. Then there's a small group where no matter what you do in those areas it still doesn't help, and that's where you can measure testosterone and see whether replacing that is a viable option. We are very careful who we choose to trial on testosterone as there's very limited long-term research in women. Sometimes the testosterone levels are fine and then you don't have other options, because there's really nothing out there that has been designed to help women specifically with sexual function, whereas obviously there is for men.

Miriama Kamo

'I've been asking myself some hard questions.'

Journalist Miriama Kamo presents TVNZ's current affairs shows *Sunday* and *Marae*. She's also a children's book author and works on a lot of other projects behind the scenes. The moment Miriama realised that she might need a little help with her menopause transition was when she yelled at a young woman in the street. It wasn't that she didn't deserve it; just that yelling isn't Miriama's normal response.

But backtracking a bit, Miriama's body had already been through a lot. She suffered endometriosis — which involves very painful periods — and the grief of several miscarriages. At the start of her forties she went into peri-menopause, and wonders if that might have been influenced by the laparoscopies she'd had for her endometriosis.

'I have to say my forties have been very hard work because of the shifting hormones,' says Miriama. 'It's also been a time when I've been asking myself some big questions. Am I who I want to be? Do I contribute enough? Am I prioritising the right things? While all these questions have been in my head, my hormones have been raging.'

Miriama experienced anxiety for the first time in her forties. She had brain fog and felt dizzy, had difficulty remembering words and never felt totally on top of things.

'Going on HRT was a big move for me, because I don't like taking medication unless it's absolutely necessary, but I thought I'd better do something,' she says.

The hormone therapy has helped ease hot flushes, but it didn't seem to touch the brain fog and the anxiety. Then Miriama discovered that she has extremely low blood pressure, which can lead to some of the symptoms she had been putting down to menopause, such as dizziness, fatigue and forgetfulness. So it's difficult for her to know which is to blame for the way she feels, or if it's a mix of both.

Overhauling her lifestyle is the way she's trying to tackle it. Miriama was already pretty healthy; she stopped drinking alcohol at age 30 and never really drank coffee. She has cut gluten, sugar and red meat from her diet, is doing yoga and has been having sessions with a breathing specialist.

'Everything at the moment feels in service of not creating inflammation that might lead to anxiety,' she says. 'I'm trying to deal with the whole thing, all at once. I feel like I've had years of eating and drinking whatever I wanted, now I just have to do things differently.'

This was meant to be the year of Miriama saying 'no', but between charity work, speaking engagements, book projects and learning te reo Māori, she has been saying yes more than she had planned.

'I was going to be a no-ninja, but I'm not a ninja at all,' she says, ruefully.

One of the talks Miriama gives is called 'The four Ms' — menstruation, miscarriage, mother-hood and menopause.

'Aside from motherhood, these are things I don't think we talk about openly, not just as women but as a society,' she says. 'And I don't know why we treat them as taboo. They're sacred experiences of womanhood and they should be celebrated and honoured that way.'

Miriama is very comfortable talking about menopause to a room full of hundreds of people. 'But the complex thing is that I haven't told my boss yet,' she says. 'My boss at work has, as far as I know, no idea.'

This might change, as she is keen to write about menopause and to continue being a part of more open conversations about it.

'At some point you have to shake hands with life and say "this is happening",' she says.

Miriama feels less invincible these days, and is more aware of time passing, which is probably what has really freighted her forties and some of those big questions that have been on her mind. Still, she is feeling positive about what the next decade holds.

'When I turn 50 everything is going to become clear again, that's what I've told myself. My memory will be sharp again, I'll run through the grass and the sky will always be blue. I definitely have this fantasy about what my fifties will be like because the forties have really whipped me.'

'He didn't fall apart because he found out there were several women in his staff that were going through menopause. It was just sort of like, "Oh well, turn the air-conditioner on." '

— *Michelle Obama on her husband, former US president Barack Obama, on* The Michelle Obama *podcast,* What Your Mother Never Told You About Health *with Dr Sharon Malone.*

Chapter 10

Food: friend or foe?

Almost all of my life, I've had a terrible relationship with food. For years I was either on a diet, or having a pre-diet binge and eating everything in sight. My mother was very aware of her weight (although she has always been reasonably slim, actually) and I remember us both joylessly eating those Styrofoam-like crackers and watery cottage cheese for lunch. I started counting calories early.

There were other influences. I watched more episodes of *Baywatch* and *Charlie's Angels* than was healthy, and thought I was supposed to grow up and look like those women. Then along came the supermodel era, and beauties like Elle Macpherson, Naomi Campbell and Cindy Crawford were our ideals. I was working on magazines by then, so had a good idea of how much retouching of photographs went on — but even so I thought my body was deeply flawed because it didn't look as taut and terrific.

I spent a lot of time in the gym doing the high-impact aerobics that are probably the reason my knees give me so much gyp today. I starved and binged through my twenties and thirties. The amount of mental energy I devoted to thinking about what I ate and didn't eat, what I weighed and ought to weigh, and the massive amounts of guilt attached to both, could have been redirected to running a small country. I loved food, but thought it was my enemy.

In my forties something changed, and I can't entirely explain why. I must have realised that I was never going to look like a supermodel. They probably didn't look like that most of the time, either, and if they did, it was because they worked at it harder than I ever could. I was always going to be curvier, but so long as I was in the healthy range, that didn't matter. Being skinny wasn't going to make me happy. Enjoying food without a side order of guilt almost certainly was.

And so I stopped dieting. There were no more forbidden foods. I haven't counted a calorie in well over a decade. I eat three meals a day and snack if I'm hungry. That's not to say I'm living on pizzas and burgers. I try to make those meals and snacks healthy ones and eat a lot of vegetables, pulses, lean proteins, nuts and healthy fats (plus butter, because what is toast without it?). I worked out that carbohydrates are my kryptonite, so I consume less and generally try to have them earlier in the day. I still enjoy beautiful sourdough bread every morning for my breakfast. I'm half Italian, so pasta and risotto are my birthright and I love them deeply. But if I have less of those things then my clothes don't start getting tighter.

It's difficult to have a conversation about weight these days without being called out for fat-shaming. To be clear, mine is not the body beautiful. I have cellulite, I wobble, and the answer to the question 'does my bum look big in this?' is a definitive yes. This is about being healthy — not about looking good or being more attractive to others. It's about staying strong and fit, because it seems to me that strong, fit women have a nicer life.

In my forties I lost a little weight, very slowly, as a result of stepping off the binge/diet cycle, cutting the excess carbs, and actually giving my body the nutrition it needed in a sane and consistent way. So I wasn't quite prepared for what would happen in my fifties. Alien fat glommed onto my body in places where there had never been fat before. My stomach blew out, my breasts got bigger, my waist thickened, and probably there is back fat there, too, but I'm too scared (and also too inflexible) to check properly.

I hadn't changed the way I was eating, but my body seemed to require less fuel than before. A friend tells me it only gets worse, and once over the age of 60 you have to choose between food and wine. She was joking. I think.

Still, it's true that post-60 the metabolism starts to

slow, and actually in a way she was right because wine is all empty calories, and if you're eating less then what you do put into your mouth needs to be nutrient-dense. I'm not talking superfoods because I don't believe in them. You can keep your crispy-dried kale and your matcha powder or whatever the latest thing happens to be. The truth is that the body requires adequate nutrition, but more of a good thing is not necessarily healthier. Every now and then you'll read about a plant food — like, say, broccoli — that contains a substance with cancer-fighting properties. But to access a significant amount of that substance by eating raw broccoli would require chewing through unrealistic amounts of the stuff.

Food can be *good*, but it's *not* super. The body needs food, but food is not medicine. Blueberries are loads better for you than biscuits, but they're not miracle workers.

One of the confusion-creators around diet is that the science can seem like it's all over the place. This is because many studies looking at nutrition are observational. They rely on people accurately recording what they've eaten. And although they can often prove a link between a particular diet and a health outcome, they can't show that the diet is a cause. A study might show that people who eat lots of vegetables live longer. But those vegetable-eating individuals might be more likely to not smoke, get loads of exercise, take supplements, have a healthy bodyweight, live in an area with less air pollution, and be affected by a number of other factors that influence longevity. And so we see conflicting headlines — like butter is good for you, butter is bad for you — because there's some science around to support both statements.

~

When I changed my ways in my forties I decided that, as much as possible, I would only eat real food. Now I'm not churning my own butter, pressing my own olive oil or even baking my own bread, because I'm as chronically time-poor as the next person. But I do try to avoid ultra-processed foods — anything with a lot of chemical additives that is over-packaged, ready-made stuff with ingredients I don't recognise on the label.

Then a few years ago I read a book called *Swallow This: Serving Up the Food Industry's Darkest Secrets* by Joanna Blythman. One of the advantages of being a freelance journalist who writes a lot about health and science is that you can track people down and interview them, which is what I did with Joanna. Afterwards I kind of wished I hadn't. It was an unnerving process shopping for food with all this new knowledge about what might have been done to it. Suddenly I found myself spooked by things I had assumed were healthy, real-food options. And I asked questions, lots of questions — what exactly had been done to this product to keep it fresh so long, why did it always appear and taste exactly the same, what happened to it before it was put into its packaging, and how safe was that packaging? The process of filling a supermarket trolley had never been so fraught.

When she was researching her book, which looked at manufactured food, Joanna blagged her way into a huge trade show in Frankfurt called Food Ingredients, which attracts thousands of producers from around the world. What she found inside the vast hall was something that looked more like a surreal modern-art installation than a food show — phials of neon-bright liquids, pyramids of powders, solutions to foam, firm, emulsify, stabilise, gel, coat and glaze, to extend shelf life, improve mouth-feel and give a fresh-like flavour.

'At Food Ingredients there was nothing you would want to eat,' Joanna told me. 'No one was eating; they all knew that was not what they were there for.'

It's much cheaper to make food filled with synthetic chemicals to give taste, texture and colour — there are big profits to be made. But how toxic is most of that cheap food? Yes, sure, we do have a comprehensive Food Standards code to control what additives can be used and in what amount. But does anyone actually know what all the many synthetic chemicals we're exposed to in every aspect of our life are doing to our bodies when they are combined together, day after day, week after week? No, they do not. No one has the full picture. And that is scary.

According to the United Nations Environment Programme (UNEP), humans use over 100,000 different chemical elements and compounds. They are in almost every product we buy — not just food, obviously — and managing them is a global problem. Our own Environmental Protection Agency is working towards reassessing a number of these, including insecticides and fungicides commonly used in our food production, because there are reasons to believe they might be harmful; but resources are limited, so it's taking a while.

Besides influencing the risk of cancer, daily repeated exposure to common chemicals may be doing everything from lowering sperm counts, triggering asthma, affecting thyroid function, disrupting the immune system and contributing to the obesity epidemic. Yes, chemicals can make you fat. Professor Bruce Blumberg from the University of California refers to these compounds as 'obesogens'. He says they re-program how our cells work in two main ways: they can promote fat accumulation through increasing the number and size of fat cells, or they can make it more difficult to lose fat by changing our ability to burn calories.

The obesogens identified so far include fungicides used on fruits and vegetables (the things we're told to eat more of to lose weight), compounds in plastic such as bisphenol A, and phthalates used in everything from food packaging to cosmetics.

'There are many sources, and trust me no one is measuring the levels of any of these chemicals in any people anywhere,' Bruce told me.

Bruce is the author of a book, *The Obesogen Effect: Why We Eat Less and Exercise More but Still Struggle to Lose Weight*. He is concerned that we're not looking at the effects of exposure to low levels of endocrine-disrupting chemicals over long periods of time. And he says that if you mix chemicals that change your metabolism with a diet that's not so good to begin with, then you have a recipe for weight gain.

There are many of areas of life where it's impossible to control exposure to endocrine-disrupters. But food, and the way we store and handle it, does give us an opportunity to do this, and the same for things like household cleaners and beauty products. Avoiding anything ultra-processed and highly packaged is a start, although I do appreciate that a lot of those fake foods are cheap and convenient, and if you're on a budget or very time-poor then they are useful.

In Bruce Blumberg's home there are no non-stick pans, stain repellents or chemical cleaners. Plastics are shunned, he avoids packaged foods and tries to eat organic as much as possible, not because it's more nutritious — although it might be — but because it's less contaminated.

Organic and spray-free food is generally pricier. You can rinse and scrub regular fruit and vegetables to try to remove some of the surface pesticide residue. A 2017 study by researchers from the University of Masschusetts[1] found that soaking apples in a solution of baking soda and water for 12–15 minutes was more effective than rinsing or using bleach. But it didn't completely remove traces of pesticide that had penetrated into the peel — the only way to get rid of that completely was to peel the apple, and then you miss out on nutrients.

I have a vege patch and am a very lazy gardener, so there's no spraying going on out there. This season, despite mostly ignoring it, I have had great success with spinach, herbs, spring onions and celery. Oh, and silverbeet. I don't think I even planted any of that, but it sprouted. It's all fertilised with rotten horse manure and compost when I can be bothered chucking some on, and eating my home-grown produce I do feel like I'm getting maximum nutrients. But if I relied on what I can grow, I would pretty much starve.

So my 'real food' philosophy is mostly around trying to avoid the stuff that's filled with additives and packed in plastic (although cheese appears to be unavailable any other way except in the fanciest and priciest of delis). I don't heat up food in plastic, because chemicals can leach out of it and into what I'm about to eat. And I've given up one-use plastic food wrap because, aside from anything else, it's bad for the planet.

I want to eat delicious, healthy food, and enough of it

to sate me — not crap and certainly not chemicals that might possibly lead to weight gain.

~

Another other reason to avoid over-processed foods is that they're believed to be addictive. The science around this is still reasonably controversial, but it makes sense. Doing a lot of the pioneering work in the area is a woman called Ashley Gearhardt. She's an associate professor of psychology at the University of Michigan where she has a lab designed to look like a fast-food restaurant.

In her research Ashley has found that some foods are particularly effective at engaging the brain's dopamine-producing reward system.[2] These are the ultra-processed foods combining sugar, fat, salt and refined carbs in a way that isn't ever found in naturally occurring food sources. She explains that our brain simply isn't equipped to cope with these products. In fact, it evolved to help us through scarcity by priming us to want exactly these sorts of high-calorie snacks.

'It used to be that the best source of sugar we had in the natural environment was a berry, or some honey that we had to scale a tree and fight bees off to get, so it was rare and not that intense,' Ashley told me. 'Because we're designed to seek them for survival, it doesn't take much for these foods to be engineered in a way that makes the reward systems go awry.'

Work by other researchers has demonstrated the effect that ultra-processed food has on the brains of animals. A study by Florida scientists Paul Kenny and Paul Johnson[3] showed that when rats were fed a diet of junk food they became hooked.

The foods that are most tied in with addictive markers are, predictably enough, chocolate, ice cream, fries, cookies, chips, cake, popcorn, cheeseburgers and muffins. Ashley's team has shown that simply looking at a chocolate milkshake activates parts of the brain that are associated with motivation, desire and drive, far more than looking at a plain glass of water.[2]

There is a *lot* of ultra-processed food out there. A 2019 'state of the food supply' report[4] produced by researchers at the University of Auckland found that two-thirds of packaged supermarket food is unhealthy. 'That's a lot,' Sally Mackay, one of the report's authors, told me. 'And half the products are discretionary — we don't need them.'

The things we've done to food in the past few decades go a long way towards explaining why the average weight of populations in the developed world has risen steadily. It makes me angry that big companies have made profits from products that have — and still are — doing damage to people's health. Walk into a petrol station, and you'll see a bank of fridges filled with sugary, fizzy drinks.

Entire aisles of supermarkets are filled with chippies and biscuits. And don't start me on the number of fast-food outlets you'll drive by on a road trip through Aotearoa New Zealand.

I don't need any of that stuff. My midlife body is losing muscle, gaining fat and gradually changing shape, no matter what I do. It's a natural process and there may be sound evolutionary reasons for it — adipose tissue is the prime source of oestrogen for the post-menopausal woman and we do continue to need it.

But women evolved to spend their middle years covering large distances on foot as they foraged for sparse amounts of food. While I sit down at my desk for long periods of time, then quickly push a trolley around a well-stocked grocery store. So I'm going to do whatever is possible to limit my exposure to obesogens and addictive junk foods if there's any chance at all that they're making the whole situation worse.

~

While I will never be skinny, I would prefer not to get any larger than I am right now, because that would expose me to health risks that are already increasing in middle age.

Having type 2 diabetes isn't fun. In this country we have a rising tide of it, fuelled in part by one of the highest rates of obesity in the world, and it is affecting people at younger and younger ages. By 2040 it is estimated that 7% of the New Zealand population will be suffering from it.

Type 2 diabetes occurs when there is too much sugar in the bloodstream. Blood sugar levels naturally shoot up after a meal as the stomach breaks down food and releases glucose. The body deals with that by releasing insulin from the beta cells of the pancreas. If those cells are compromised in some way and fail to make enough insulin at the right time, then diabetes develops.

To make matters worse, in type 2 diabetes the body doesn't respond well to whatever insulin is on offer. In the long term this has devastating health consequences as the body's network of blood vessels gets damaged, creating nerve problems that result in amputations being necessary, and leading to sight loss, heart attacks, strokes, kidney damage and early death. What people with type 2 diabetes are typically offered is a steadily increasing amount of medication, some of which causes further weight gain, and eventually insulin injections.

It's not related to the way you look. Scientists have discovered that having lots of fat beneath the skin isn't the cause of type 2 diabetes. The problem is tinier deposits of what is known as 'visceral fat' in the liver and pancreas. As little as half a gram of fat inside the pancreas prevents the beta cells from manufacturing and releasing insulin. So people can look skinny on the outside but be fat on the inside.

Visceral fat is also associated with increased risk of heart attacks and strokes, as well as widespread inflammation that can affect things like the liver and joints. And guess what? During the menopause transition, women are more prone to gaining visceral fat. This is why our risk of developing type 2 diabetes suddenly increases at this time — we're about three times more likely to have it than we were before.

Do scientists know exactly why? No, of course not. But as well as the fall in oestrogen, there is a drop in sex-hormone-binding globulin (SHBG), a protein that carries both testosterone and oestrogen. It seems that if you're already overweight, the impact of this may be greater. And it's also possible that the drop in oestrogen leads to an increase in appetite, so we've got another perfect storm brewing.

HRT can help. Putting some of those hormones back in keeps cholesterol and visceral fat under control and improves insulin sensitivity. Obviously that goes hand-in-hand with diet and lifestyle — it's not going to make up for mainlining on carbs, fat and sugar.

What if you already have type 2 diabetes? Well, there's some good news. Roy Taylor, a professor of medicine and metabolism at Newcastle University in the UK, has long been working on a non-drug answer to the problem. He's shown that it's possible to put it in remission purely by losing enough weight. His trial, DiRECT,[5] run through

GP surgeries in the UK, saw almost 50% of participants reversing their diabetes and able to stop taking medication. They did it by eating 800 calories a day for two months, often living on liquid meal-replacement drinks.

Shoot me now! If I tried that approach, I know it would destroy my fragile but happy friendship with food; I'd be back to bingeing and starving in no time. And I don't want to go back there. Diabetes prevention is one of the reasons why I'm trying not to gain any more weight. But if you're already there, and your blood sugar is out of control, then Roy Taylor does make a strong case for his horrible calorie-restricting diet.

'If people lose 15 kilos within six years of being diagnosed, they've got a nine-out-of-ten chance of getting rid of their diabetes,' he told me. 'And if they lose 10 kilos they've got about a two-thirds chance. Once you go beyond ten years it's not impossible, but it's much less likely that diabetes will be reversed.'

Roy's theory is that every individual has their personal fat threshold — the point at which no more fat can be taken into the layer of cells under the skin. It has to go somewhere, so ends up not only inside the tummy cavity but also inside the main organs of the body. How early this happens is determined by genetics, and Roy is pleased that this theory has taken some of the blame away from the body-shaming weight debate.

'When I explain the personal fat threshold to patients

in the clinic, I get this profoundly relieved reaction,' he says. 'I think it's something important to shout about.'

Ethnicity seems to play a role. Roy Taylor and his team have shared their expertise at scanning the pancreas for fat with New Zealand researchers who are working on the High Value Nutrition project, and looking at the underlying causes of type 2 diabetes, how to diagnose risk earlier, and the optimum diet to prevent it. Sally Poppitt, the University of Auckland professor leading the study, told me that the scans show Asian Chinese people are more at risk having fat in their pancreas compared with Europeans. The other groups at higher risk for type 2 diabetes are Asian Indian people and anyone with a family history of the condition.

To reverse type 2 diabetes and become drug-free, the speed of weight loss isn't important — just that you get below that personal threshold and stay there. Roy Taylor describes alcohol as liquid fat, which is something I try not to think about as I enjoy a glass of wine. And he shared one more interesting thing — after you've lost weight, you're likely to need only around three-quarters of what you used to eat.

One of the reasons that people find it so difficult to maintain weight loss is that their resting metabolic rate (RMR) has changed. RMR determines how much energy we burn simply to stay alive — to keep our hearts pumping, our digestive systems working, our lungs breathing. With weight loss, RMR slows. This phenomenon is known as metabolic adaptation. It acts to counter weight loss and is part of the body's defence system against possible famine.

A scientist called Kevin Hall at the National Institutes of Health in the US led a really interesting study to show how the body works to return to a set point with weight.[6] He followed fourteen contestants from season 8 of TV's *The Biggest Loser*, measuring long-term changes in their RMR and body composition. Kevin discovered that the RMR of contestants was substantially reduced after the competition, and it was still low six years down the track. People were burning around 500 calories a day less than expected given their age and body composition. Not surprisingly, many had regained a substantial amount of their lost weight.

But wait, there's more. Not only had their energy expenditure decreased long-term, but changes in hormone levels conspired to make these ex-contestants hungrier. Leptin, the hormone that makes you feel full, declines with weight loss, and in *The Biggest Loser* contestants it never fully returned to its original levels. So essentially they were fat again, even hungrier than before and burning fewer calories.

~

All of this stuff seems like a lot of bad news, but it does appear that maintaining a healthy microbiome can make a difference. The microbiome is the colony of bacteria that lives in your gut, around 30–40 trillion microscopic creatures that interact with your body systems in complex and still largely mysterious ways. Since the middle of last century we've been slaughtering them with antibiotics and starving them out with ultra-processed foods, and it is possible that this has contributed to everything from rising rates of type 2 diabetes to irritable bowel syndrome, depression and anxiety.

Microbial restoration is one of medicine's new frontiers, and microbiome sequencing is all the rage. You can buy an at-home test kit, check your poo and discover what your balance of good and bad gut flora is looking like. But with any diagnostic test there are two questions I would always ask. First, how reliable is it? (And who knows at this point with these tests?) And second, will the results change the way I behave?

Whatever the composition of your poo, it makes sense to eat a gut-flora-friendly diet and that's one with lots of whole fruit and vegetables, fermented foods like sauerkraut or kefir, low sugar and no artificial sweeteners, no junk . . . oh, and apparently some seaweed. Microbes also need resistant starches from plant fibres that the body can't digest. Sources include onions, leeks and garlic, as well as witloof and endive, Jerusalem artichoke, asparagus and green bananas. Fun fact: if you cook and cool potatoes, pasta, garden peas, beans and lentils, then you'll significantly increase the amount of resistant starch in them.

There is no perfect way of eating that suits us all. We're not identical machines, and our microbiome is likely to play a big part in that.

Tim Spector, professor of genetic epidemiology at King's College London, has done some really interesting work with twins. In the PREDICT I study[7] he gave hundreds of twins identical foods and found that their bodies behaved differently. There was an eightfold difference between individuals — normal people eating the same meals — in terms of their metabolic response, and he believes that the differing microbiome is a reason why.

So if your weight is creeping up, it isn't necessarily that you are greedy and consuming too many calories, says Tim. The real problem is that the one-size-fits-all dietary advice about calories, fats and carbs doesn't allow for this individual effect. That and the fact that the food industry has been persuading us into eating ultra-processed rubbish for several decades.

The future is personalised nutrition. In the meantime, Tim suggests aiming for the diversity of having 30 different plant foods a week. 'Too many people get stuck in a rut and have a banana a day. And when you are shopping, avoid anything that says low-fat, sugar-free, added vitamins, etc. Go for quality foods that are going to help your gut microbes.'

I may not believe in the magical healing powers of food,

but I don't think there is any doubt that a bad diet can be destructive. And actually there *is* some evidence that tweaking your diet in midlife can help menopause symptoms — like that observational 2019 Japanese study that suggests upping vitamin B_6 (found in a variety of foods including beef, salmon, tuna and chickpeas) and oily fish can reduce the severity of hot flushes.[8]

Phytoestrogens are another food often touted as meno-pause-friendly. Contained in soy products like tofu, they are believed to be the reason why Japanese women complain less about hot flushes. Most research has failed to come up with solid evidence that phytoestrogen supplements or foods can have an impact on menopausal symptoms.

The reason may be that a lifetime of eating these foods makes the difference. Or the microbiome may be involved. It could be that Japanese women have a genetic advantage and can convert the compounds in plants into something useful for the body. Or it may even be a cultural thing — perhaps Japanese women are more reluctant to mention their hot flushes.

While we know that these plant compounds do interact with oestrogen receptors, and that they can mimic or interfere with the hormone, it is taking a while to work out how we can harness this. There is some emerging science that how you consume soy may make a difference. A small study published in the medical journal *Menopause*[9] found that eating half a cup of whole soybeans every day alongside a low-fat vegan diet reduced moderate to severe hot flushes by 84%, and in more than half the women in the study they disappeared all together. Many participants also reported differences in sexual symptoms, mood and energy. A few noticed weight loss and better digestion. Researchers believe that this effect is due to the production of a non-steroidal compound called equol, which is produced when soy's isoflavones are metabolised in the gut as part of normal digestion. This could be a game-changer, and who doesn't love edamame beans?

~

I think the take-out message from all of this for midlife women comes down to the 'real food, mostly plant, not too much' advice from American author and journalist Michael Pollan. There is an entire industry conspiring against us, and for the good of our health we have to resist the palatable, addictive foods they want to sell us. Because potentially they are worse for us at this stage of life than ever before, with our arteries more likely to harden and our blood sugar more likely to spike and our bones more likely to crumble and our brains fog. This is a time to nourish our bodies with good-quality food, not chemical-laced crap. Eating well is one of the foundations of self-care that will keep us healthier in midlife and heading towards older age. It's also a reliable source of everyday pleasure.

Being free of the guilt and obsession around food, and able to revel in its deliciousness, is one of the best things to have happened to me in midlife. It turns out that food isn't my foe; it's a friend I love and need, but only in moderate amounts.

Q&A with Christchurch dietitian Sara Widdowson of Mission Nutrition

Do we need to eat differently in midlife?

A woman's nutrition needs change throughout her lifespan. The work I do with clients in menopause is often around discussing the weight gain that happens. It's to do with the reduction in oestrogen, which drives insulin resistance in midlife women and means they're more susceptible to that ease of weight gain and difficulty shifting weight, particularly in the central torso area. The little tricks they once used, like eating less bread or having less wine, don't work anymore.

What does work?

With my clients I use a moderate lower carbo-hydrate approach to help combat insulin resistance — so not keto. It's still important to eat enough. The big mistake I see clients make is that they eat fewer calories than I would feed a toddler. They significantly drop their energy intake, trying to lose weight. That makes the mood side of menopause even more difficult to handle, and also slows down the metabolism. So I get them to reduce the starchy white carbohydrates and increase the protein and colourful vegetables.

What if you're vegan or vegetarian?

Pulses like lentils, beans and chickpeas are both protein and carbohydrate. So you need to be conscious of that and have a bit less rice on the side, or perhaps choose lower-carbohydrate vegetables like pumpkin and carrots rather than potato. But you can also get protein from tofu and fermented soy like tempeh, or eggs and dairy if you're vegetarian.

Any nutrients you need to be sure to step up?

Magnesium is important for sleep. You can take a supplement, but I would also make sure you get plenty in your diet — it's in things like dark chocolate, nuts and seeds, dark leafy greens and whole grains. Another thing I talk to clients about is that oestrogen has a protective effect on cholesterol levels, and we lose that advantage in menopause. I'll walk them through cholesterol advice —

reducing saturated fat, limiting takeaways, eating lots of fibre and lean proteins. We'll also have a conversation about eating for bone strength, so getting enough calcium and vitamin D.

Do caffeine and wine become more problematic for our bodies in midlife?

What I see a lot in clinic is that women aren't sleeping because of the hormonal impact on insomnia. They use caffeine all day to pick themselves up and alcohol to wind down at night. What they don't realise is that alcohol has a similar impact as caffeine on sleep. There's also evidence that it affects dopamine activity in the brain. [When we drink, the brain's reward circuits are flooded with dopamine, which produces the buzz. But over time, alcohol can cause dopamine levels to plummet, leaving you feeling miserable.] Also alcohol and caffeine are vasodilators; they dilate blood vessels. If I've got clients who struggle with hot flushes, I'll ask them to do an experiment where they reduce the grog and the caffeine for four weeks and see if they notice any change in their symptoms.

Can you limit midlife weight gain?

It's very individual, and there is obviously a conver-sation around what is a realistic goal. If a client was trying to be the same size and shape they were at 22, we would talk about body acceptance. Also discussing the hormonal changes invites self-compassion. This change of shape is part of the normal progression in life and it's important to make peace with that. But absolutely you can control the weight gain trajectory by making some changes. That might mean exercising because it makes you feel good and helps with blood pressure, rather than punishing yourself trying to shift those extra couple of kilos.

~

Dame Hinewehi Mohi

'I wasn't feeling like myself.'

Dame Hinewehi Mohi is a softly spoken woman. Chatting via Zoom with Hinewehi in her Hawke's Bay home office, I found her a considered and thoughtful person. But I also know that she is a powerhouse. A singer and songwriter, in 2004 she founded the Raukatauri Music Therapy Centre, inspired by her daughter Hineraukatauri, who has severe cerebral palsy. The organisation has gone from strength to strength since then, helping thousands of New Zealanders.

When she was 46 Hinewehi had breast cancer, needing a double mastectomy and chemotherapy, as well as a long course of the drug tamoxifen, which blocks the effects of oestrogen in the breast tissue and causes menopause symptoms.

'Because I was so wrapped up in my breast cancer treatment and feeling pretty awful with the chemo, especially towards the end, I didn't really think too much about menopause,' she says. 'I can't really remember having bad hot flushes.'

The cancer treatment was successful, and in the decade since Hinewehi has been grateful for her good health. But more recently she has sensed a mental shift.

'About six months ago I started to feel as if I was losing confidence and my mood was quite down,' she explains. 'Generally I'm an upbeat person and I wasn't feeling like myself.'

One area where Hinewehi had lost confidence was with her singing. She doesn't perform much in public these days, and if asked she tends to suggest a younger singer in her place.

'My voice isn't the same,' she explains. 'I don't have the same control over it and I think the tamoxifen treatment might have affected my vocal chords, which is why I weighed up the risks and decided to discontinue it. In the five years since, I'm not certain if menopause has specifically caused further issues, or if it's just the physical changes brought about by ageing generally.'

With a busy work life and her daughter, now in her mid-twenties, needing support, Hinewehi had been feeling overwhelmed. She wasn't sure whether this general sense of anxiety was a result of living though a tricky year with the Covid-19 pandemic. At a scheduled check-up with her breast specialist, she mentioned how she had been feeling and the doctor, suspecting that it might be due to her time of life, suggested she take anti-anxiety medication. That has proved to be a good move and, while she expects only to need the extra help temporarily, it is definitely helping.

'It's really helped to level out my feelings,' says Hinewehi. 'Before it felt like a roller-coaster.'

It can be difficult to talk about how you're feeling, particularly as this sense of anxiety and lost confidence tends to come on gradually. So Hinewehi hopes that sharing her experience will help others going through the same thing to feel a little less lonely as they try to decide how best to deal with their symptoms.

'I think it's important for people to know that someone who appears to be managing her life isn't always on top of everything,' she says.

In her mid-fifties, Hinewehi is busy as a trustee of the music therapy centre and in her role with APRA AMCOS developing Māori music. These are her passions as well as her job and they continue to drive her.

'I know some people aspire to retire as early as they can, but I don't want to stop doing this kind of work until I really can't do it anymore.'

Chapter 11

Out of our way, we're coming through

When I was young, I was raped. A man broke into the house where I was living and I woke to find him lying on top of me with something sharp held to the side of my face. For a few terrible moments I thought I was going to die. Afterwards, when it was all over, I called the police. As they were driving me to the police station, I heard one of them saying on his radio: 'Yes, we've got the victim with us.' From the back seat of the car I piped up: 'I'm not a victim.'

And then I piped down again, as it occurred to me that they probably thought I was strange. But, against all the odds (rape examinations were traumatic in the 1980s), I continued to feel that way. I hate the word 'victim'. It's destructive, it robs you of power and dignity, it's a terrible word — I chose to be a survivor.

Re-framing it that way helped me in the weeks and months that followed. I was 21 and had just finished university. I was determined not to allow this stranger to turn me into someone who went through the rest of her life scared.

All these years later, I'm still careful about making sure doors and windows are locked before I go to bed. I prefer to sleep beside a burly husband and at least one large dog — good luck getting past them. Yes, I'm careful, but I haven't let what happened stop me having adventures, or travelling alone, or making new friends, or trusting people. Because I'm *not* a victim.

I bring this up now because I worry that there is a risk of menopause making victims of us. While in the grip of sweats and flushes and sleeplessness and uncontrollable moods, it can feel like a calamity. It's easy to focus only on the negatives. So I'd like to re-frame this time of life: we're not victims, we're survivors.

I'm wary of being too ra-ra about this life stage. All the 'you are woman, you are in your power, you are fierce and free and renewed' stuff is too simplistic — and also unhelpful if you happen to be having one of those days when you feel like a wet noodle. For the same reason I've had to unfollow a lot of midlife Instagram influencers. Seeing them doing handstands while wearing bikinis got a bit dispiriting, as it didn't bear any resemblance to my everyday life.

I want to keep it real here. I don't want to make anyone feel left out or inadequate. But at the same time, we need to smash some of those tropes to smithereens. Tropes like menopause is an illness, it's a crisis, a time to dread, the end of what makes us women, the onset of invisibility, something to endure in silence and shame, your best years are behind you, your currency is lost. All of those tropes.

~

In her book *The Change*, feminist writer Germaine Greer called menopause 'the antechamber of death'. Well, the life expectancy of a woman in Aotearoa right now is 83.5 years and if you consider that the average age of menopause is 52, that's an extremely spacious antechamber right there. (Wāhine Māori and Pasifika women have lower life expectancies than Pākehā and Asian women. While this is an inequity that needs to be addressed, they do still have many years to enjoy post-menopause so let's not hear any more about the antechamber of death, please.)

And there is good stuff coming. When I asked women to share some of it, I heard about increased energy and post-menopausal zest. Many seemed to be exploring their creative side and taking back ownership of their time after years of giving it to others. These were the true freedom years, women told me. Not your twenties, when you're busy building yourself from the ground up and trying to forge a career and relationships.

This is what they said some of the good stuff was:

Freedom. Finally fully free of caring about what others think. Free of being sexualised. Free to redefine myself.

Financial security, resilience, perspective, perseverance. Have time to lead a healthier lifestyle. Also it's been many years since I was last sexually harassed by randoms on the street.

I'm pretty fearless these days. I like that a lot. Hot flushes are power surges and I use my awake patches in the night to plot revolution.

I love having no periods, and all that comes with it. I walk past the tampons/pads in the supermarket and just smile that that's not part of my world.

Dressing to please yourself and not the trends. Not being cold in winter. Not giving any fucks. Body acceptance and love. No periods. No need for contraception. Better sex because of it. More money. More-secure life.

Time for yourself.

Many women said that grandchildren were a joy in this stage of life. And looking after mokopuna is apparently what nature intended us to be doing around about now. It's called the grandmother hypothesis. The reason women evolved to stick around for so long after our ovaries have been decommissioned is thought to be a human baby's need for a lot of care. Compared with other species, it takes us humans ages to get up on our feet and attain any level of independence.

And that is why a middle-aged female is quite a human thing to be. Until recently it was believed that the only other mammals to live for decades after menopause are toothed whales, like orca. Now giraffes are believed to spend up to 30% of their lives in a post-reproductive state. That is likely to be for a similar reason. It's an advantage to have an older, wiser female to share the burden. They are repositories of knowledge, skilled at finding food — whether that's a whale hunting salmon, or an early human foraging for berries, or a giraffe seeking the tastiest leaves and buds. No longer bothered by periods or pregnancy, these elders can devote the rest of their days to caring for their children's offspring.

Grandchildren do sound great — all the fun of kids without the stress of being the one responsible for keeping them alive on a daily basis. But there are many women who long for a family, try everything, and can't get pregnant. And some, like me, who choose not to. The grandmother hypothesis implies that we no longer have a purpose and that we're living those extra 30 years just to grow hairs on our chins and gain extra belly fat. Clearly this is *not* the case.

Killer whales and giraffes might be leading the same existence that evolution shaped them for, but we humans have changed things up a bit. Today's generation of older women, more educated and experienced than any who have gone before, exposed to feminism and attuned to the idea of having it all — these women might not be so ready to glide gracefully into a middle age composed of grandmotherly duties, good works and a bit of gardening. They're thinking about second careers, new challenges and awfully big adventures. Some women are powering up at a time when they might be expected to start planning their retirement.

In 2021 global media company Forbes named its first-ever female 50 Over 50 Impact List[1] — entrepreneurs, leaders, scientists and creators who are achieving their greatest accomplishments and making an impact in the second half of their lives. It included Kamala Harris, who at 56 became the first woman, first black American and first Asian American to hold the office of vice president. TV producer and screenwriter Shonda Rhimes, 51, who smashed Netflix records with her show *Bridgerton*. Nancy

Pelosi, who became America's first Speaker of the House at 66. And Julie Wainwright, who survived the crash of her business Pets.com and at 53 started again, founding luxury online consignment store The RealReal, which, in 2021, Forbes said was worth $US1 billion.

We don't have a 50 Over 50 in Aotearoa New Zealand yet, but we ought to, because here too there are plenty of women who are older, wiser and bolder — like Vanessa Sorenson, who grew up in a trailer park, left school at sixteen with no qualifications and by 50 was head of Microsoft New Zealand. Kelly Martin, 53 and head of our biggest TV production company, South Pacific Pictures. Annabel Langbein, running a foodie empire at 62. Helen Clark, at 71 working with global organisations for gender equality, climate action and pandemic preparedness. Carmen Parahi of *Stuff*, who at 51 is leading the way in changing how Māori are represented in our media. Patricia Grace and Fiona Kidman, both still writing in their eighties.

I'm not saying that every woman has to be boldly succeeding and achieving. But I do think it's time to change the narrative about menopause. It's not a demise, it isn't a fading away, and it certainly isn't the antechamber of death.

~

On the Menopause Over Martinis Facebook page (sign up, it's great) I came across this post by Wellington woman Gabrielle Martell-Turner, and I loved it so much that I messaged her straight away to ask for permission use it in this book. She agreed. This is what she wrote:

> *I am finally admitting that I adore being enraged. Rage is getting me where I need to be. I'm full to the fucking brim with peri-menopausal rage and I'm using it. Menopause is still such a taboo. As is being REAL about the grief of ageing. It's like any transition, but it's an ending, and endings are raw, tough and painful. I'm ripping my way out of my old skin, clawing, roaring, crying and it's snotty, messy, and 100% fucking graceless. I was swimming this morning in Lyall Bay. Well, swimming is not quite the word, being blown over the waves, knocked off my feet and my togs kept falling down. I got pebbles in places pebbles have no place being. It was also exhilarating. It was a real-life metaphor for the wild, uncontrollable ride that is ageing. I do a huge amount of self work, so I understand everything I'm going through. It's glorious in the same way that any death or transition is glorious. In a rage-fuck kind of way. In a roaring, ugly, bursting out kind of way. Being down here with my beautiful daughter is so bittersweet. Loving that I have raised such an adventurous soul, and mourning her three-year-old self at the same time. I'm two years away from*

being the age my mum was when she died, at 54. She never had this chance to age. I'm grateful for my life, I'm grateful that I'm the sort of kick-ass woman who swims in the Wellington sea in July, and I'm also full of such conflicting, hormone driven emotions that it's sometimes hard to see straight.

Thanks, Gabrielle. Nothing on earth would get me to swim in Lyall Bay on a winter's day, but I'm with you every step of the way otherwise. It truly is a wild ride, this menopause transition — there's a lot of snot and tears as well as rage and sweating, but there are gifts, too, and the rage might even be one of them. If — rather than clenching our jaws — we harness that fury and use it to get where we need to be.

My husband's favourite book is the *Road Code* (true) and he quotes from it a lot, generally when I'm driving. I always reply that in New Zealand there is really just one rule of the road, and it's 'Out of my way, I'm coming through.'

That's exactly how I feel about my life right now: 'out of my way' because I don't have time to waste, I'm all out of patience — there are things I need to do, and 'I'm coming through'.

Since I arrived in midlife, I care much less about being liked and I'm not so concerned with being lovely. The unnecessary niceness has leached out of me along with my hormones. I don't have time to waste being pointlessly polite to people who don't deserve it.

We women are meant to be lovely, aren't we? We're not supposed to be demanding, or shrill, or pushy or bossy, or we'll pay. It has been that way for centuries. Gregorio Marañón, a pioneer of endocrinology in Spain in the 1900s, held the view that a woman's temperament determined her menopause experience. The virile, bold and energetic woman would suffer more, he claimed, than the very womanly woman who is delicate, fragile and childish. In other words, 'Be lovely or you'll pay for it.'

This attitude lingers on. Women in power, especially politicians, know all about it. In the final debate of the 2016 US presidential election, Donald Trump leaned into the microphone as Hillary Clinton spoke about social security and called his opponent 'such a nasty woman'. The phrase inspired a movement. It became a hashtag, an international rallying call for feminists; and you could even buy a Nasty Woman T-shirt — celebrities like Katy Perry and Julia Louis-Dreyfus sported them.

Trump tried the same sort of put-down with US vice president Kamala Harris. He called her 'totally unlikeable'. Well, if you're unlikeable because you fight for what you believe in and you smash glass ceilings and you don't ever let yourself be bullied, then sign me right up.

I may not be very lovely these days, but it doesn't mean I'm going around being randomly unkind and unpleasant. It's just that in the process of growing older and wiser, I've realised that loveliness isn't mandatory and it isn't always helpful. I don't have to prove myself anymore. If people disapprove of what I say or do, I don't have to care. I feel freer to be myself even if that self is sometimes quite spiky.

'You know they all hate you,' my husband said of a particular group of (inconsiderate) people.

'That's fine,' I replied. 'I don't like them much either.'

Mostly I keep a lid on my 'unloveliness'. I go about my everyday life playing nicely, but still it's there, bubbling under, ready to spurt out like a lahar if I'm provoked. There are times when you have to speak your mind — times when it's important. There are times when you have to say 'Out of my way, I'm coming through.'

I've also acquired something I call 'the menopausal glare'. It's a look that says more than words ever can, and can repel a man at twenty paces. Some years ago, when I was still quite lovely, I saw this in action for the very first time. I was at a party and being harassed by a very drunk guy. Try as I might to get rid of him, nothing worked and he kept leering and breathing his stinky vodka breath all over me. Finally I sought refuge with an older woman. 'Help,' I pleaded. 'I can't make him leave me alone.' She said nothing at all. Instead, she unleashed a glare. It stopped him in his tracks; he withered visibly, and then he backed away. It was magnificent.

Now I, too, have the power of the menopausal glare. It arrived out of nowhere one day and I'm making the most of it. Loveliness is over-rated. Well, it is if it leads to us putting up with things when we shouldn't, to being downtrodden, abused or overlooked. Or even prey to persistent, vodka-breathed creeps at parties.

Auckland social anthropologist Jane Horan says that the menopause is as much cultural as it is biological. We've been sold this idea that it's a goodbye to everything you hold dear and a stretch of barren years ahead. I think we need to use our rage to fight against that. When I met her in an Auckland café, Jane told me that while she wasn't having a particularly difficult menopause, she was crushed by the idea of turning 50 and began to wonder why. She started to realise that it wasn't so much what was happening to her body that bothered her, but Pākehā *society*'s view of what it means to be an older woman. By 'society' what she essentially means is the patriarchy — all those men who for hundreds of years have been telling us that menopause turns us into hairy-faced unfuckable viragos.

'It has taken me a while to realise that menopause isn't just a set of symptoms, it is also a whole lot of baggage that is foisted on me, upon all of us,' wrote Jane in a thought-provoking piece for online magazine *Ensemble*.

We've been made to feel like victims of our time of life, told we're a set of symptoms and there's nothing to be done about it, instructed to shuffle off into invisibility and settle into the La-Z-Boy of life, that we're un-gendered, hags, crones, past it — or (if we dare to look youthful) that we're cougars.

Women are starting to bring about a change. There are midlifers on TikTok railing against invisibility. There are a lot of stroppy memes — like 'One of the best things about getting older is knowing someone is an asshole before they even speak' — and an array of podcasts and blogs. There is coverage in women's magazines, talk on radio, a TV documentary (UK presenter Davina McCall's *Sex, Myths and the Menopause* which you can watch on YouTube) and lots of books. In fact, the menopause memoir is becoming an actual genre.

After fifty-plus years of feminism, it's about time we stopped letting ourselves be dismissed and diminished. Out of our way — we're coming through.

We are not *exiting* womanhood, just moving to another stage of it. This is a transition, a shift, and like any change it can be challenging at times. But there is no need to suffer, as symptoms can be managed. And some day you're going to emerge out the other side.

'The menopause comes and it is the most wonderful thing in the world,' says Kristin Scott Thomas's character in the TV show *Fleabag*. 'And, yes, your entire pelvic floor crumbles, and you get hot and no one cares. But then you're free, no longer a slave, no longer a machine with parts, you're just a person, in business . . . It's horrendous, but then it's magnificent. Something to look forward to.'

So many women I've spoken to see menopause as a blessing. I've discovered that this is your moment to reinvent yourself after years of focusing on the needs of everyone else.'

— *Oprah Winfrey, in her own magazine.*

Chapter 12

I want to feel like a natural woman

As soon as I started researching this book, which involved a lot of googling and joining social media menopause groups, my screen lit up with adverts aimed at midlife women, most of them trying to sell me a hailstorm of supplements. To swallow so many pills would be a full-time job and keep my liver and kidneys very busy processing it all. Curcumin, red clover, pine bark . . . I was bewildered. I was also rolling my eyes so much that I thought they might have to be surgically returned to their rightful position. The power some people have given to the word 'natural' is disturbing.

So let's be clear: it is natural for hormones to decline.

Hot flushes are natural. Those sudden brain zaps of electricity? Weird, yes, but also natural. What we're looking for is something in nature to help us deal with all that. Not all the things at once; ideally just one or two and in an effective dose.

Stick the prefix 'Meno' in front of anything and it confers the power to appeal to a lot of midlife women. MenoMe, Meno-Free, MenoCalm, Meno Magic, MenoCool, Menopace, Menosan. I'm not saying that none of them work, but I would question how much evidence there is that some of them do, and also how you're meant to choose between them.

~

First of all, though, we need to go into the world of bio-identical hormones and it's a fraught space. When the WHI study (see page 109) frightened the life out of everyone and doctors were scared off prescribing HRT, it left a lot of women high and dry. They were still having a really bad time. And they still wanted help. There was a large gap in the market, and bio-identical hormones leapt in to fill it.

Bio-identicals were marketed as being natural and therefore safer. They're not made by Big Pharma but by smaller compounding pharmacies, and have a 'bespoke' element to them. All of that was very appealing, particularly to a modern breed of privileged, dynamic women who were used to taking control and practised at problem-solving. This seemed like the obvious way to deal with the problem at hand.

Compounding pharmacies had been around for ages. Their job was to tailor-make a prescription medication to suit an individual's needs. Say you were allergic to a carrier ingredient in a particular drug — lactose, maybe — then the pharmacist could make you up a lactose-free version. When bio-identicals came along, suddenly there was a lucrative new line of business for compounding pharmacies.

Let us be very clear: bio-identical hormones are still synthesised in a lab. They are still active with a potential for side-effects. Natural doesn't necessarily mean safe.

And there are a number of other concerns. Compounding pharmacies don't have the same controls and regulations as the makers of pharmaceutical medications do. There is no guarantee of a consistent dose, or even consistent ingredients. There are no requirements around testing, safety data, or reporting of adverse effects. There have been cases where hygiene measures in compounding labs haven't been stringent enough and products have become polluted with bacteria or fungi. In the US back in 2012, contaminated steroids from a compounding centre resulted in an outbreak of fungal meningitis and a number of deaths.

Endocrinologist Anna Fenton says that for a while, even in New Zealand, it was a bit of a Wild West affair with people being prescribed hormones purely on the basis of a telephone consultation and having a package couriered to them.

The Australasian Menopause Society is very clear about its position on compounded bio-identical hormones: not recommended, not safe, no more natural than HRT, and they've been associated with endometrial cancer because the dose of compounded progesterone wasn't strong enough to be protective.[1]

I can see that in the days when the only choice was oestrogen extracted from mares' urine, going down the bio-identical route seemed worth it, even if it was much more expensive. But now oestrogen patches funded by Pharmac are plant-based and body-identical. And now we can access oral micronised progesterone that is molecularly the same to the hormone our body is missing. And we can get free blood tests rather than paying out for saliva or dried urine tests. My feeling is that bio-identicals may have had their day. Certainly I dislike the element of privilege that their price tag brings in a country where we actually do still have affordable, often free, healthcare.

Having said all that, I've spoken to women who used the progesterone cream approach (so no oestrogen) and say that it helped with bloating, breast tenderness, mood swings and sleep. So, if you can find a reliable source — like a holistic GP — who can advise you whether it's appropriate and prescribe a dependable product, then it's an affordable option that you might want to trial. But it won't protect your womb from the risk of endometrial cancer if you're also taking oestrogen.

~

The 'wellness' industry is huge, and researching the various charges for women wanting to 'balance their biochemistry' I was shocked at some of those prices — in some cases, thousands for testing and an individualised lifestyle programme. There is always someone trying to part you from your money, and in menopause that seems particularly true. As journalist Suzanne Moore says in her *New Statesman* essay 'There Won't Be Blood', 'It's a minefield of wishful thinking.'

Some things are not worth bothering with. Cross yam cream off your shopping list. It may contain diosgenin, the substance that is chemically converted into progesterone, but your body cannot do the converting by itself. One study of 23 women who used it for three months found no side-effects but little effect on menopausal symptoms either — it worked as well as the placebo.[2]

Lack of evidence is the problem with so much complementary and alternative medicine (CAM). Either no studies have been done, or only a limited number and not especially high-quality. More research is definitely needed.

The Cochrane Library (see the end of the book for the web address) is a useful place to look for information. It's an international not-for-profit with lots of open access online, and there is a plain language version of each article. What Cochrane typically does is examine all the available research and come up with a conclusion.

Take black cohosh, for example. A plant related to the buttercup family, preparations made from its roots and stems were traditionally used by Native Americans, and today it is the most common botanical that women take for menopause support. Cochrane looked at sixteen studies involving 2027 women, and found insufficient evidence to support its use. However, the reviewers said that there was adequate justification for further research.[3]

Part of the reason for that justification is that there are some clinical trials that support black cohosh. One 2018 study of 80 post-menopausal women compared it with evening primrose oil, and found that it was more effective in reducing the number of hot flushes and improved quality of life.[4]

Black cohosh also seems to be reasonably safe. There were reports of liver damage, but it's thought that this might have been due to contaminated products, and the most common side-effects reported are stomach upsets and rashes.

A brand of black cohosh sold under the name Remifemin is one for which there's good anecdotal evidence, and several women told me that it helped them through the worst of their flushes. 'If it works for you, it really works,' said one. It's been around a long time and clinical trials spanning several decades have found that it can be helpful to ease hot flushes.

On balance I would say that black cohosh is worth a try while we wait for the scientists to (hopefully) play catch-up and find out more. You want to make sure you buy good-quality supplements, with an effective dose, and you might choose to see a registered medical herbalist to see if it, and other botanicals, are appropriate for you.

One of the advantages of alternative therapies is the amount of time practitioners give you. GPs have limited time. Increasingly they seem to be trying to move us out of their waiting room and on to Zoom or telephone consultations, which is apparently the way ahead in a country where, according to a survey by the Royal New Zealand College of General Practitioners[5], almost a third of doctors intend to retire within five years, almost half within ten, and 31% rate themselves high on the burn-out scale. This is a system under severe stress.

In contrast, Jessica Giljam-Brown, the medical herbalist I chatted to, lavishes an hour and a half on consulting with a new client, and then there are follow-up emails at least three times a week afterwards. Naturopaths who I spoke to said the same. That sense of being listened to, and the holistic approach rather than looking at one symptom at a time, is a wonderful thing. Fifteen minutes with a harried GP just doesn't compare.

It shouldn't have to be an either/or situation. Conventional and alternative medicine can work hand- in-hand, and it's possible to find practitioners from both sides who will collaborate. Surely that's the ideal, as herbs are potent compounds and some might be unwise to take alongside other medications or conflict with an existing health condition.

'Most of my patients use a combination of hormone therapy and natural treatments,' says Christchurch naturopath Lara Briden. 'And they get better results than they would have with hormone therapy alone.'

If you do want to experiment by yourself, Lara has published an excellent book called *The Hormone Repair Manual,* which is a good place to go for guidance. She lists supplements, what they should be used for, and trusted brands. Lara told me that she doesn't like the idea of being a 'gatekeeper' to the world of natural therapies and there are plenty of safe and affordable things you can try. Topping her list are magnesium, taurine and glycine to support the nervous system and help with hot flushes and sleep problems.

The North American Menopause Society (NAMS) has a long position statement on non-hormonal management of hot flushes, which you can find online.[6] As you'd expect, there's a lot of 'not finding enough evidence' going on.

- Exercise, yoga, avoiding triggers — all get a resounding 'we don't know'.
- NAMS found that cognitive behavioural therapy reduced the severity of hot flushes but not their frequency, and says that it's an effective treatment for breast cancer survivors who are unable to take HRT.
- There is a small, statistically insignificant amount of evidence that mindfulness helps.
- Hypnosis seems more promising, as there is some evidence that it reduces flushes, improves mood and helps sleep, but acupuncture doesn't have much to support it.
- According to NAMS, evening primrose is ineffective, flaxseed (a.k.a. linseed) is safe to eat but it's not going to stop you flushing, ginseng doesn't help, and maca root has

had some interesting results but the trials were small and poorly designed.

- Antioxidant-rich pine bark is one that has a small amount of interesting evidence to back it. While an effective dose hasn't been established, it does seem to improve symptoms, and the brand that was evaluated, Pycnogenol, did seem to improve symptoms.
- Pollen extract looks promising.

There are plenty more things to try — curcumin, turmeric, red clover, chaste berry — as well as a lot of products that use doses of different botanicals in combination.

Cannabidiol (CBD) is also having a moment. Recently there has been a surge of interest in its use for lots of things, including menopause. CBD is one of the active ingredients of cannabis, but taken by itself it doesn't produce a euphoric high. There are cannabinoid receptors in the brain and other parts of the body that are involved in things like mood, sleep and memory, and the theory is that the fluctuating then lower levels of oestrogen in menopause may disrupt this system and so CBD oil could reduce symptoms.

Overseas there are all sorts of CBD-laced products available — CDB tampons, anyone? — and Brooke Shields has talked about using a CBD oil on her face. In this country

CBD products are prescription-only, and at the time of writing only a few oils are approved. I chatted to Dr Waseem Alzaher at the Cannabis Clinic, and he said that CBD is particularly beneficial for managing anxiety and sleep, so if those are the things you are mainly struggling with it may be worth trying. The oil is easy to take — you just drip some into your mouth — and Waseem tells me that side-effects are rare. But it costs several hundred dollars a month, so the cost is going to be prohibitive for many.

None of the midlife women I encountered were using CBD; still, it's relatively early days for New Zealanders. In other countries the situation is different. In Canada, where cannabis has been legalised for a while, one in three women use it to manage menopause symptoms according to a 2021 study from the University of Alberta presented at the NAMS annual meeting.[7] The most widely cited reason was sleep issues, followed by anxiety, muscle and joint aches, irritability and depression.

~

Opponents of alternative therapies can be very fixed in their ideas. And it is true that there are snake-oil salespeople out there. But my feeling is that if something is safe and affordable, then there's no harm in trialling it — whether that's a herb or acupuncture. Hot flushes are only one of many menopause symptoms, after all, and some treatments may provide benefits for the sleeplessness and mood swings that can bother a woman just as much — St John's wort, for instance, which Cochrane has found is helpful to treat mild to medium depression. Or ashwagandha (*Withania somnifera*) extract, which has some evidence to support it as a stress reliever and cortisol moderator.[8]

Someone in my household (not me) has a habit of buying supplements but never taking them, and thus an entire shelf of my pantry is crowded with jars of stuff to support gut health, control stress, optimise the immune system, etc. For them to work, you do actually have to swallow the things. I'd be wary, though, of trialling too many at once.

Another caveat is that more doesn't necessarily mean better, especially when it comes to nutrients. The body can only absorb so many vitamins; then it has to store them in fat or pee them out.

Oh, and I do have a cautionary tale. A friend of mine took herself off to a naturopath when her periods stopped in her late forties, as she wanted herbal support to help her through what she thought was coming. The practitioner prescribed a few supplements but, since some weren't safe to take in pregnancy, instructed her to take a test first. Sure enough my friend was wonderfully and unexpectedly pregnant. This tale has a happy ending as she had a longed-for baby. So I would suggest identifying exactly which journey your body is taking you on, before you start ingesting anything.

Aside from that I think everybody should be allowed

to treat their menopause symptoms how they like. If you really want to put a magnet in your knickers to balance your nervous system or a jade egg in your vagina to strengthen your pelvic floor, balance your hormones and intensify your orgasm then, evidence-based or not, I don't think anyone has a right to stop you.

Q&A with Auckland medical herbalist Jessica Giljam-Brown

If I came to see you saying I was having a difficult menopause, what would you do?

It would depend on what stage you were at. You have to remember this whole menopause transition is gradual. It starts from around the age of 35. That's a time when women are often busy with career and family, and they don't notice the problems that start to creep in. Then in their forties they may become more aware that things are changing. And by 55 they may be having the hot sweats and the brain fog. Usually it's not necessary to do a lot of tests; we look at the symptoms or use blood tests from the GP. If a woman is having very severe symptoms and needs a quick fix, then typically I'd look at using HRT alongside natural therapy and work with the client's doctor or refer her to an endocrinologist. It's important to start with diet first, looking at increasing fibre and supporting healthy clearance of oestrogen, as well as blood sugar management. Most women have increased insulin resistance in peri-menopause and menopause, which can lead to low energy, mood swings, brain fog and weight gain — so I will typically do a lot of work in this area.

There are so many herbal and nutrient supplements out there, how do women know where to start?
They don't! Many women who come to me are taking the wrong things and potentially making symptoms worse. Or they're spending a lot of money on supplements that are low-dose or have ten different herbs combined in one little pill so the dose they're getting isn't therapeutically active. And the important thing to remember is that your menopause journey changes. You can't pick a supplement and be, like, yep that's me for the next five years. You need different things. There's no magic pill, unfortunately. A good practitioner will be able to assess your symptoms and prescribe herbs or nutrients that suit you at that time.

Have you got any star performers, though?
Definitely. Magnesium is a go-to. It's safe, afford-

able and works on the nervous system, so helps with many of the issues that crop up in menopause, such as not sleeping and insulin resistance. That and zinc would be the two I use the most. Then I'd look at things like taurine and glycine, which also help the nervous system and sleep. Problems with sleep are very common for women between 35 and 60, and I might also use herbs like passionflower or valerian.

What about for women who are struggling with emotional problems, loss of confidence, etc.?

I might suggest St John's wort or lemon balm, which are anti-depressant and anti-anxiety. We can also use a product called SAM-e [S-Adenosyl methionine). I find that really powerful for women who are feeling super-flat or have lost confidence — they're often the women who are getting very tearful at work suddenly. Black cohosh can help as well, which is another one of those traditional menopause herbs, and one of the reasons I like it for mood, energy and confidence support is that it helps to keep serotonin in circulation for longer, similar to St John's wort and your standard anti-depressant drugs.

If you're going to invest in supplements, is it also wise to consult a professional to make sure you're getting what you need?

Absolutely, a medical herbalist or a naturopath, or even a nutritionist who's not working with herbs can still use nutrients. It's definitely worth the cost of a consult and getting proper-quality supplements rather than taking a hit-and-miss approach, and not really knowing if what you're taking is right for you.

~

Sarah Gandy

'It affects everything about your day.'

Sarah Gandy is a radio host and has the personality to match — bubbly, upbeat, warm, fun. She was 36 when she found a lump in her breast and things got very serious. What followed was a mastectomy, and months of chemo and radiation. Sarah also had injections of the hormone-blocker Zoladex (generic name goserelin) to stop her ovaries producing oestrogen, and that threw her into an intense medically-induced menopause.

'The hot flushes were horrendous,' she recalls. 'There were nights I'd be sitting on the couch and my face would go bright red and I'd feel like my head was on fire. The only thing you can do is try to cool yourself down until it stops, so I always had a rosewater spray in the fridge. The best money I spent was at Kmart on one of those cooling pet beds to sleep on, and I had a USB fan clipped to my bedside that I'd point at my face all night long.

'Then, of course, after the hot flush comes the cold flush and you're freezing. It's no wonder that part of menopause is people who've never had a mental health problem in their life battling with mood swings. Your hormones are all over the place, and if you're not sleeping well your body doesn't know which way is up.'

Now on tamoxifen, the symptoms are less intense, and if Sarah eats well and avoids coffee, she seems to be able to avoid hot flushes — although she still sleeps with her bedroom at 19°C, meaning that her partner has to snuggle under extra covers.

Sarah will be on tamoxifen for a decade, and when she stops, she's likely to at some point go through a second, more natural menopause.

'I feel like I've had a peek into the future, like I pulled back the curtain for a little bit, and OMG it affects everything about your day,' she says. 'There were clothes I got rid of because I thought I'd never be able to wear them again; they were so hot and restrictive. A once cosy sweater became a death trap.'

When she was going through the worst of her symptoms, many people were uncomfortable and cringed if she mentioned it. 'I was the one with the horror stories and I think there was a real taboo about it.'

The whole experience has made Sarah realise that in the male-dominated world of radio, there must be many midlife women who are quietly going through the same thing.

'All these women who are phenomenal at what they do are having to keep this thing secret for fear of someone judging them or assuming they've lost their edge,' says Sarah.

Chapter 13

Hearts & Minds & Bones

We women are not the same as men. This won't come as a huge surprise to anyone at all, but, despite that, women tend to get the same health advice as men unless it's to do with our specific lady-parts. Historically, a lot of clinical trials were done using male participants because our hormones made things too difficult and messy for researchers, which means that a lot of modern medicine has actually been designed for men. This is changing, thankfully, but in the meantime we're still living with the results.

For optimal wellness, our differences are important to consider throughout our lives — and in midlife particularly so. This is because those hormones have had a protective effect, and when they disappear it can be damaging for our health unless we're careful.

I don't know about you, but I'm not interested in slowing down at this point in my life. I don't intend to shuffle off in my slippers to the sofa with a cup of tea and the *Coronation Street* compendium. I want to ride horses, and hike the Great Walks, and cycle rail-trails. My peers are paddle-boarding, kayaking, going to gigs, returning to education. One midlife former dancer I know just performed in a ballet.

You need good health for all of that, a strong mind and a strong body. And in menopause you have to work a bit harder for those things. This chapter is headlined *Hearts & Bones & Minds* because these are three key areas that we need to focus on so we can keep tramping and dancing and swimming our way to old age. That's not to say the rest of the body isn't important — top-to-toe it can give you trouble — but you have to start somewhere, right?

Hearts

Pre-menopausal women have an advantage over men, as oestrogen has a protective effect on the heart. Once the ovaries have ceased production, though, that advantage disappears. Our metabolism starts to change, body fat increases (particularly around the torso), blood pressure rises and so do low-density lipids (the 'bad' cholesterol).

Also, the speed at which our arteries stiffen up accelerates during the menopause transition. It is believed that this is because the hormonal changes result in inflammation and affect vascular fat deposits. Women who sleep badly seem to be the worst affected when it comes to vascular stiffness.

And so our risk of cardiovascular disease rises sharply with the onset of menopause. And about a decade afterwards we've caught up with men, but not in a good way. More than 50 New Zealand women die each week of heart disease, making it the single biggest cause of death for women in Aotearoa.

When women have heart attacks, they don't always experience them the same way that men do. Rather than the classic symptom of crushing chest pain, they might have less obvious signs — feeling a bit off-colour or dizzy, tired, breathless, very fatigued, sweaty or nauseous. It can be easy for women and their doctors to miss what is happening.

Gerry Devlin, a Gisborne cardiologist and medical director of the Heart Foundation, told me that women are also less likely to ask for help. He says that's because we're busy, and often focused on caring for other people. But I also suspect that women who have experienced menstrual cramps or PMS or childbirth are conditioned to doing a lot of soldiering-on, and that's why it is easy to miss the signs.

While we've seen a dramatic reduction in heart attack deaths over the past 50 or so years, there are still a large number of people who don't even make it to hospital. Gerry says that often when you talk to patients in coronary care units after a major cardiac event, they'll say they hadn't been feeling well for a while and should have seen a doctor earlier.

So a focus for the Heart Foundation is to get people — all people — to pay attention to what their bodies are telling them. If it's not normal for you, if it's been going on for a while, if there are a few odd things you've noticed lately, if things are harder to do than before, if you're experiencing a little chest discomfort — don't soldier on, but get yourself to a doctor.

In midlife you'd be wise to schedule a heart check. Your GP will do this; it involves having your blood pressure taken, your cholesterol measured, getting an HbA1c test to measure your blood sugar and see if you have diabetes, as well as going through your family history and discussing smoking.

All that information is put into a calculator — the PREDICT tool developed by University of Auckland professor of epidemiology Rod Jackson — which estimates your risk of a heart attack or stroke over the next five years. Once you know this, you can think about doing something about that risk, whether it involves improving diet, taking some exercise, losing weight, giving up smoking or going on medication to control blood pressure or cholesterol.

Gerry says that blood pressure control is one area where we could be doing better. It's a risk factor not only for stroke, but also for coronary artery disease, heart attacks and heart failure.

For women, smoking presents an extra cardiovascular risk; possibly because nicotine in our bodies is metabolised faster. Having had gestational diabetes or pre-eclampsia during pregnancy, or suffering from polycystic ovary syndrome (PCOS) may also up the risk later in life.

The Heart Foundation advice is:

- Women without any known risk factors are advised to get a heart check from age 55.
- Women with known heart disease risks should go from 45.
- Māori, Pasifika or South Asian women are advised to go from the age of 40.
- People with severe mental illness are advised to go as early as 25 (their mortality rate is two to three times higher than the general population, and cardiovascular disease is a major contributor to that).

Keeping a heart healthy is about consistency — eating well and exercising regularly in the long term — although it's almost never too late to make improvements in both those areas.

On the website My Menopause Doctor, Louise Newson (the UK doctor I mentioned earlier in the book who is a strong advocate of HRT) writes that hormone therapy has been shown to reduce future risk of cardiovascular disease when taken within 10 years of menopause. She says that avoiding HRT in menopausal woman can actually be detrimental to their health, and that the presence of cardiovascular risk factors — such as high blood pressure — isn't a reason to say no to hormone therapy, although obviously those risks should be controlled with other medications.

'The menopausal period and early menopause are an ideal opportunity to assess cardiovascular risk, and women should often be considered for HRT at an earlier stage in order to gain maximum cardiovascular protection from taking HRT,' sums up Louise. 'Women with POI [premature ovarian insufficiency] and women within 10 years of their menopause can potentially gain significant improvements in their cardiovascular health, as well as their general health, by being offered HRT. It is of utmost importance that health-care professionals are educated properly regarding the potential health benefits to be gained by taking HRT. I totally agree with the notion of encouraging as many women as possible to consider HRT as a treatment to reduce future cardiovascular disease.'

In the 1991 Nurses' Health Study, women aged 30 to 63 on oestrogen therapy had a reduced risk of coronary heart disease.[1] And a more recent study involving more than 400,000 Finnish women found that the risk of cardiac and stroke death rose in the year following HRT being discontinued, particularly in women under 60.[2]

Still, for most medical practitioners in New Zealand, heart health won't be considered the primary reason to give a menopausal woman hormones or to keep her on them. Statins and blood pressure medication are much more likely to be offered.

Even if you are on HRT, it makes sense to lead a heart-healthy lifestyle, consuming healthy fats like nuts, fish and avocado rather than saturated fats, cutting down on salt, having lots of fresh fruits and vegetables. That, plus being active and not smoking, is pretty consistent health advice for anyone at all these days. Having had a time with no kitchen when we ate a lot of takeaways, the other thing I would say is that home-cooked food is almost always healthier than anything an Uber Eats driver brings to your door.

Minds

My mother-in-law has dementia. It's been a slow process, thankfully, and she's held onto her personality. She's still a lot of fun, has retained an ability to enjoy life, even though it's very restricted now, and is often very funny. She remembers who we all are, still recalls a lot of family history and knows exactly what her favourite shade of lipstick is — MAC Morange. But ask her what she had for lunch, or even where she is right now, and she won't be able to tell you. Her ability to make new memories is failing her.

The latest research suggests that these changes possibly started happening decades ago, and there may have been a window of chance when her fate could have been changed.

Women's brains age differently to men's, and menopause plays a key role in this.

In midlife a woman's brain is remodelled. We know this thanks to a neuroscientist called Lisa Mosconi, who is the director of the Women's Brain Initiative at Weill Cornell Medicine in New York. She did a study where she scanned the brains of more than 160 women who were at varying stages of the menopause transition, looking at things like structure, blood flow and energy, and did the same thing with men in the same age group.[3] What she found was that in the women the brain changed a lot, but not in the men.

Our brains and our ovaries are part of the neuro-endocrine system (a messenger system in the body involved in the release of hormones) and so they 'talk' to each other constantly. Oestradiol, the form of oestrogen that we lose in menopause, is important for energy production in the brain — it pushes the neurons to burn glucose and create energy. So once the levels of this hormone decline, brain energy drops; it slows down and ages faster.

What those scans showed was, during peri-menopause, women lost brain cells that processed information along with the fibres that connected those cells. Hello, brain fog — that's where you came from. No wonder so many of the women I spoke to had been through a stage of fearing that they had early-onset dementia. It also explains why a survey by the UK's Nuffield Health organisation found that one in four women with menopause symptoms were concerned about their ability to cope with life.[4]

Post-menopause, that loss stops. Researchers believe that the brain goes through this process and then regroups as it adapts to the new normal. So it is highly unlikely that you're getting early-onset dementia. However, during peri-menopause those women who have a genetic risk factor for Alzheimer's begin to develop amyloid plaques. Not everyone with plaques goes on to have dementia, but the plaques are a feature of the disease and so personally I'd rather not have them.

More than two-thirds of those diagnosed with Alzheimer's are women. Historically we've been told this is because we live longer, but it is becoming apparent that there is more going on. It is believed, for instance, that oestrogen influences the way the body makes antioxidants, protecting the brain cells from damage, and so hormone therapy may be beneficial. Oestrogen also influences the way brain chemicals such as serotonin and dopamine are used to send signals.

Some encouraging research has come from the University of Arizona.[5] It found that women on hormone therapy were up to 58% less likely to develop neurodegenerative diseases, including Alzheimer's and dementia. The type of HRT the women took made a difference — those using body-identical oestrogen and progesterone (like the Estradot patches and Utrogestan capsules commonly prescribed in New Zealand) had a greater reduction in risk than those taking synthetic hormones. Also, the protective effect was greater for those taking the therapy for more than a year.

This is significant because previous studies have delivered mixed results — most likely because much of it has been focused on women who took the older styles of hormones. In fact, ten years on, the participants from the WHI study (see page 109) actually had an *increased* dementia risk (and yes, scientists are still following and studying that original group of women). That might partly be due to the type of HRT — they were taking oestrogen synthesised from mares' urine — but again, it seems that timing is crucial and the window of opportunity to gain benefits is around menopause, not much later.

As I write this, HRT is still not recommended for dementia prevention because — as usual — more research is needed. But if you have a family history of dementia, you might not want to wait around for the science to get definitive. Brain protection certainly deserves a place on that list of risks and benefits that midlife women are making.

~

Again, it's worth saying that HRT isn't the whole outfit, merely an accessory; there are lots of other things we can be doing to preserve our brain power for as long as possible.

In 2020 the *Lancet* Commission on Dementia announced that 40% of cases could be prevented or delayed if twelve risk factors were targeted over a person's lifetume.[6] This group of world-leading experts advised that higher education levels, social contact and physical activity all reduced the risk of dementia. Meanwhile, factors increasing our chances of developing it early were midlife hearing loss, traumatic brain injury, high blood pressure, diabetes, excessive alcohol consumption, obesity, smoking, depression and air pollution.

There is masses of science to prove that exercise — particularly exercising the brain and the body together — is vital for the brain. This is one area at least where no more research is needed. Movement, it seems, is the real miracle pill. Food also has a role to play, with the Mediterranean diet the real star again, although basically any low-processed diet rich in lots of colourful vegetables and fruits, good fats (so those from plant sources), fibre and lean protein is good.

Lisa Mosconi advises getting enough fluids, as the brain is 80% water and every chemical reaction in it depends on that water to occur. Dehydration causes the brain to shrink, which is hardly going to help the fog situation. For many of us, everyday life is dehydrating. We spend a lot of time indoors, sealed in our cars, homes or offices, under hot lighting and surrounded by electronic devices.

The conventional wisdom is that eight glasses of water a day will see us right, but this advice appears to have no real basis in science. It seems to date back to 1945 when the US Food and Nutrition Board recommended that people consume 2.5 litres of fluid a day, adding a significant — but largely ignored — coda that much of this quantity could be found in foods.

Rehydrating does *not* mean constantly sipping water. There are lots of water-rich plant foods like cucumber, celery, apples, iceberg lettuce and leafy greens — all excellent when blended into a green smoothie. Soups and bone broths count as fluid, as do things like herbal and fruit teas, and soaked chia seeds. Eight glasses of water a day won't do you any harm, but whether you actually need it is questionable.

Anything that keeps the body healthy is going to be good for the brain. Risk factors like not getting concussions and looking after our hearing are things we have a limited amount of control over. Two areas where we *do* have more sovereignty are education — it's never too late to return to some form of learning — and social connection. When the pandemic lockdowns limited my social connections, I realised just how important those catch-ups with friends were for my wellbeing. It doesn't really surprise me that they were also good for my middle-aged oestrogen-deprived brain.

Bones

Half of all women will have a fracture between menopause and the time they die. That's a lot of women. In midlife this is painful and inconvenient; later on it can be an absolute game-changer. About 40% of elderly people who fracture a hip are left unable to walk properly, many won't get back their previous level of independence, and a significant number will die within a year.

In menopause as oestrogen levels start to dip, women lose bone density; with men this bone loss happens more slowly and later. Plus women tend to have smaller, thinner bones in the first place, putting us at higher risk of the brittle-bone condition osteoporosis.

Bones might seem solid things, but like any living tissue they are in a constant state of flux. Cells called osteoclasts break down the bone's matrix of collagen and minerals, releasing calcium into the bloodstream for re-use in other parts of the body. And another set of cells, osteoblasts, balance this out by forming new bone. The entire skeleton renews itself within 8–10 years.

With age, things change. For the first twenty years of life our bodies build new bone more quickly than the old bone is removed. By age 25, most of us have reached our genetic peak bone mass. Later in life the process is reversed: bone is broken down more quickly than it is formed.

Osteoporosis isn't inevitable, but there are a host of factors that increase our chances of developing it — such as a poor diet, a sedentary lifestyle, smoking, excess alcohol and coffee intake, family history, being underweight and taking certain medications like the glucocorticoids used to treat asthma. However, the two most important factors are age and gender.

Calcium has long been seen as the key to keeping bones strong. Cheese, milk, yoghurt, sardines, sesame seeds, almonds — the mantra was consume plenty of these sources of calcium throughout your life, and get enough vitamin D to aid its absorption. We were all told that in older age you should increase your intake of both, possibly with supplementation.

Then a team from the University of Auckland shook things up with a review study published in the *British Medical Journal*.[7] They found that increasing calcium intake, whether through diet or supplements, was unlikely to improve bone health or prevent fractures in older people. Not only is a high calcium intake not a sure-fire winner, but excessive supplementation has been associated with gastrointestinal side-effects and kidney stones, and may even be detrimental to cardiovascular health.

The same team found that taking vitamin D supplements wasn't helpful for boosting bone mineral density or preventing fractures, either, except in rare cases where lack of daylight is a factor (such as elderly people who don't get outside much, or women who always keep their face and body covered).[8]

That doesn't mean that cheese and sunshine aren't important — you do need adequate amounts of both — but more of them isn't better.

~

So what *can* you do?

Well, in midlife — particularly if you've had a fracture — it's not a bad idea to make having a DEXA scan part of your body maintenance plan. This is a quick and painless low-dose X-ray that will measure the bone density in your spine and hip. You'll get what is known as a T-score, which compares your bone mass with that of a healthy young adult. If the score is low, then you may be at risk of developing osteoporosis.

There are lifestyle measures you can take to protect bone health — the usual quitting smoking and decreasing alcohol consumption are right up there. There's also good evidence that too much caffeine is damaging. Researchers from the University of South Australia found that high doses (800 mg) of caffeine consumed over a six-hour period almost doubled the amount of calcium lost in the urine.[9]

That's about eight cups of coffee, which is more than most of us would drink in a day. The participants actually chewed a caffeine gum rather than swigging a lot of flat whites, but when you think that you also find caffeine in energy drinks and tea, it starts to seem easier to overdose.

Plus, of course, you do need to make sure you get enough vitamin D. This is present in some foods, but the bulk of it is synthesised in our skin when we are exposed to sunshine. Only around 5% of adults in this country are deficient, but a further 27% have below the recommended level according to figures from the Ministry of Health.[10] As well as being essential for the health of our bones and teeth, vitamin D has also been linked to everything from better brain performance to improved cardiovascular health, a lower risk of cancer and a stronger immune system.

The need to expose our skin to sunshine is complicated by the need to protect it from damaging UV rays. The advice is to improve intake by exposing large amounts of skin — so your arms and legs rather than just your face — for a shorter period of time. In summer this should be done before 10 a.m. and after 4 p.m. And in winter during the middle of the day. There isn't an exact prescription for the length of exposure required, as lots of factors come into play, including skin pigmentation, your age and your location.

Food sources of vitamin D include oily fish, dairy, eggs and fatty cuts of meat, but if you are deficient then diet alone won't improve your status. If you are concerned about vitamin D levels over winter, you can request a blood test at Labtests without a GP referral, although there is a small cost.

If your bones turn out to be worryingly weak, there's a medication called zoledronate or zoledronic acid, which can be given by an infusion every eighteen months or so and has been shown to reduce the risk of fracture. Other drugs from the same family — known as bisphosphonates — can be taken as a pill. But there is also evidence that our skeleton can be strengthened with exercise.

Not just any old exercise, though. In her LIFTMOR study,[11] a team led by bone expert Belinda Beck of Australia's Griffith University showed that high-intensity loading is required — so this means lifting heavy weights or doing jumping exercises.

As Belinda said when I interviewed her, some women never lift anything heavier than their handbags, and if you want to grow bone then your handbag isn't going to cut it. She has devised a programme, Onero, that's available online, and she says that as well as bone strength it will also improve general strength, balance and posture. But if you'd rather go it alone, then blending weight training that targets major muscle groups with impact training like jumping, rope-skipping or hopping plus a balance exercise such as tai chi is ideal. Going for a walk isn't so effective unless you make it harder for yourself by incorporating some jumps.

'Anything that keeps you active is better than doing nothing,' says Belinda.

The average woman loses up to 10% of her bone mass in the first five years after menopause. So to get maximum benefit for osteoporosis prevention, HRT needs to be started soon after menopause. The Australasian Menopause Society says HRT reduces the rate of spinal and hip fractures by 40%, but that it's most useful in women under 60. If you stop taking HRT, then bone mineral density will start to decline, and so women who are at fracture risk should go onto other medication.

There is a form of HRT called tibolone (brand name Livial) which is a synthetic steroid molecule that your body breaks down to make hormones. This has been found to be effective in the prevention of bone loss, but it doesn't seem to be as helpful for hot flush control as standard HRT and there are concerns around cancer risks — ovarian, breast and womb — as well as stroke risk. It's not funded in New Zealand and, although it is available on prescription, doesn't appear to be used much.

Also, your doctor is unlikely to prescribe HRT purely to boost bone density, because at the moment, in this country at least, it's considered to be an additional benefit rather than a primary reason to give hormones.

In the UK, where the menopause revolution is happening faster and more furiously, there is pressure for the focus to widen from vasomotor symptoms — flushes are just one aspect of menopause, after all — and for the power that treatments have to improve other aspects of health to be considered. Bone health is another area where more research probably isn't needed — there have been lots of studies that show HRT helps.

So when you make your HRT pros and cons list, particularly if you have a family history of osteoporosis or you've had a scan and got a low T-score, I reckon you're going to be inking this in high on the column of pros.

Q&A with endocrinologist and coach Sasha Nair

As a coach and a hormone specialist, what's your advice to empower midlife women through this change?

If you feel you may be suffering from symptoms of peri-menopause or menopause, it is a good idea to see your doctor to confirm the cause of your symptoms and discuss options for treatment. There are medical options available to help, and if the initial medication regimen doesn't suit you (or if once you're feeling better you feel you no longer need it), the medication can be adjusted, changed or tapered off under the supervision of your doctor. Yes, having symptoms is a natural part of the transition to menopause for some women, but it's helpful to arm yourself with the information to weigh up whether or not using medication is right for you.

Taking a broader perspective, midlife is also a great moment to take stock of your general health and mindset. This can be a really busy time with career, family commitments and other demands, and it is more important than ever to make time for self-care. Sleep, nutrition and movement is not only good for your health and performance but also for your ability to cope with stresses on a day-to-day basis, so do see your doctor if symptoms are interrupting your sleep. Often as women we feel guilty taking time out for ourselves, but prioritising self-care is a necessity if you want to feel, look and function at your best, and be able to optimally serve others.

Self-care in terms of our mental and psychological health is also important. Our mindsets and beliefs around the changes of midlife can affect how we experience it. When you embrace each stage of life, the benefits that each stage brings, and focus on being the best version of yourself at that particular stage, you may have a different experience than if your thoughts instead centred on dreading getting older!

There is evidence that mind–body approaches such as cognitive behavioural therapy can be helpful for mood symptoms, anxiety, sleep and even hot flushes and sweats. Other mind–body practices that you may like to try include meditation and yoga.

There is probably a complex interaction between the physiological changes of peri-menopause, physical symptoms and mood, so I think optimising your general and psychological health and reflecting on your mindset and beliefs around midlife, even before you have symptoms, may be of benefit in helping you through the transition.

What's your approach with HRT?

My approach is very much tailored to the individual. I take into consideration which symptoms are present, how troublesome they are, any pre-existing health conditions and the woman's preferences. We discuss the pros and cons of treatment options, and decide together on the best treatment regimen to start on. From there, it is not unusual to need to tweak the regimen if the symptoms haven't improved satisfactorily or if there are side-effects. After that, review at least annually (whether with me or the GP) to see if the treatment is still appropriate and whether it is still needed. Coming off medication is usually a gradual taper.

So generally I avoid a blanket approach or saying 'everyone should do this', and advise women instead to see a physician experienced in menopause management who will work with them on an individualised treatment.

Chapter 14

Why OK Boomer is not OK

In the midst of the sweeping of floors and the loading of dishwashers, the cycles of laundry and the hauling of bags of groceries back from the supermarket and turning them into meals, while all that normal everyday stuff was going on and as I was trying to work out who I was going to be when I was properly grown-up, I got old. What the actual *fuck*?

It took me ages to realise I wasn't young anymore. Literally even my chin had got old, and I was still swanning about thinking of myself in much the same way as I ever had. It shook me when the truth dawned. It's still shaking me.

Middle age is incredibly hard to define. You're not

young anymore, but nor are you elderly. It's like being mid-Pacific on a flight from Auckland to Los Angeles. You're not in either of those places, but you are somewhere. Unhelpfully, there is no reliable yardstick to measure when midlife actually starts. Back when three score years and ten was considered a decent innings, it fell at 35. The *Oxford English Dictionary* says it kicks off at 45, and for women menopause is often used as a dividing line.

No one wants to be old, do they? Ageism is the last bastion of allowed prejudice. In this newly woke world, thankfully it's not acceptable to shame people because of their gender, skin colour or body size anymore, but unfortunately it still seems fine to age-shame a woman.

That's why dropping the 'M-bomb' into conversation is so taboo. Being menopausal is a clear identifier of oldness. So don't talk about it with your colleagues, in case they think you're past it and irrelevant. Don't talk about it with your partner or your friends, because it's a buzzkill. Have your hot flushes quietly and out of sight. Keep a stiff upper (preferably plumped-up) lip on those mood swings. Plaster yourself with products that have the words 'anti-ageing' on the jar, even though we all know that if any of those youth potions did what they claim on the label nobody would have a single wrinkle.

It's as if by getting middle-aged we've done something embarrassingly predictable and deeply uncool. While being old is unavoidable if you live long enough, looking your age actually isn't 100% obligatory these days. There is no end of cosmetic 'tweakments' available if you've got the time and money. Botox, fillers, lasers and lights, facial peels and facelifts. If it helps you get up in the morning and face the world, and you're not living on two-minute noodles in order to pay for it, then go for it, I say. I'm all for freedom of choice.

Still, I'm a little concerned at the way some Hollywood stars are eradicating even the subtlest signs of the passing years from their faces. A few are so smooth now that they look like eggs with features. I'm particularly worried about Nicole Kidman. At this point she seems only capable of one expression, a slight pout. I'm sure she thinks she's conveying emotion — she is an actor, after all — but it isn't translating to actual facial movement due to expertly paralysed muscles.

It's not only Nicole — there are plenty of other Hollywood women who aren't letting age so much as caress a cheek. Julia Roberts, Jennifer Aniston, J.Lo, Angelina Jolie, Sandra Bullock, Halle Berry. Recently I saw a shot of Sarah Jessica Parker and Kristin Davis on the set of the latest *Sex and the City* reboot. They had boosted their lips and hardened their expressions so much that they didn't look old, but they didn't look young either — they just looked 'other'.

Watch pretty much any American movie or TV show, and it isn't hard to spot an ageless wonder. It strikes me that there is something sinister going on. Nicole is in her fifties, so isn't she permitted a few wrinkles, a subtle softening of the jaw line, a slight thinning of the lips, a few signs that she is ageing? Male actors are allowed to get saggy, baggy and wrinkly, after all — have you seen Hugh Grant recently? — so why aren't their leading ladies?

~

I do sympathise with any woman trying to make her way in an industry where she's not supposed to look a bit frayed around the edges. But I also hate the tyranny of it, and the sexism and ageism; the idea that we have less currency if we've let ourselves look older. Should we have to be so well preserved? We're women, not marmalade.

For this to change we need more role models like Helen Mirren, Meryl Streep, Michelle Obama and Kate Winslet. Women who possibly may have tweaked a few things here and there, but can still look happy, sad, shocked or angry as the situation requires.

It's practically a political act to let your hair go grey these days. Women are called 'brave' if they start to silver. That seems ridiculous, because it shouldn't require courage to show the world that you're ageing.

We need to use some of that menopausal rage to fight against the idea that it's shameful or a failure to age. Let's change the way we talk about it, too. Past your use-by date, over the hill, old dear, senior . . . ugh. Don't euphemise me — just call me old, because that's what I am and it shouldn't be pejorative.

I am on the cusp of Boomer and Gen X, although I don't know who decides these things or even why they bother. When you are on the wrong side of a generation gap, you suddenly realise what a nonsense it is.

OK Boomer is *not* OK, because age has nothing to do with attitude. Boomers fought for gay rights and women's rights, battled racism and apartheid and nuclear bombs, struggled for abortion rights and cannabis reform. They fought for the environment, too. They didn't succeed, but they did try — Greenpeace was founded in 1971 by people who are old now; Sea Shepherd was started in 1977. Those people didn't hit middle age and immediately start voting against drug reform and denying climate change. Yes, there are reactionary and unreconstructed Boomers — but age is not the determining factor.

You can say there's always been intergenerational friction, that's just how it ever was. But that's like saying there's always been racial segregation, or unequal pay for women, or homophobia, and, oh well, what can you do? Sometimes things have to change, and the tension between young and old is one of those things. Because it's bad for everyone.

I don't lack the thought power to understand what younger people are going through. I *can* appreciate the pressures. I worry about how they're going to afford to pay off their student loans and buy a home. I'm concerned about the planet not being hospitable enough for them to live on. The negative power of social media, the rise of anxiety, the way globalisation might rob them of jobs — that's the content of many a 3 a.m. panic and dread session, and I don't even have children of my own.

I care about younger people, I'm interested in talking to them and understanding their perspective, I like having them as friends, but in return I'd prefer it if they didn't take one look at my crinkly face and make a whole bunch of assumptions about me. Dismiss me, dislike me or deride me if you want, but *not* on the basis of my age.

Because I'm going through a few things, too, actually.

Menopause is sometimes referred to as 'like a second puberty', and I suppose it is in terms of being a hormonal storm. But when you're reversing out of fertility rather then heading into it, what lies ahead is something very different. You aren't on the brink of endless possibility anymore. Time is in shorter supply. It is running out. Very often my 3 a.m. panic and dread is all tied up with that. Have I done everything I should have? Been to enough places? Are there things that will never happen now? I'm over halfway through my life and I can hear doors slamming. I might never learn to speak another language fluently or travel through India or win an Oscar for best screenplay. The possibilities have shrivelled along with my skin.

As US comedian Cathy Ladman says, 'Menopause is a lot like adolescence except without all that life ahead of you.'

Doing the midlife maths is daunting. In a minute I'll be elderly; in a few more I'll be gone and someone will have to work out what to do with my surfeit of cookery books, the jumper my mum knitted me when I was 21 and a lot of heated hair appliances. Mortality is feeling very, very real.

Am I having a midlife crisis? I hope not, because it seems clichéd, risible and self-indulgent. It smacks of privilege and not having any proper problems. But I do think about that famous Steve Jobs quote from the speech he gave to Stanford University graduates back in 2005: 'Your time is limited, so don't waste it leading someone else's life.' And I do wonder: is this the right life? How did I get here? Were turns taken that took me to the wrong destination? Is there still somewhere ahead where I could make a U-turn?

Actually I doubt it, as writing is the only ability I have. My waitressing career ended after I tipped salad over a woman's head, and I was fired from a job as a shop assistant (also clumsiness-related) after being told I didn't have what it takes. Career-wise there were never a lot of choices open, and now there are even fewer.

Being middle-aged is life-limiting, and that's official. A 2014 ageing workforce survey carried out in New Zealand found that one in three employers and employees believed there were issues with age discrimination in their industry.[1] Employers say it becomes a problem at 53, while employees reckon 50. Two in five older workers said that they had experienced age discrimination in the past five years, which ranged from reduced access to promotion, to being assigned less-interesting tasks, bullying and exclusion from social activities. The Equal Employment Opportunities Commissioner at the time, Jackie Blue, reported job applicants being told 'We thought you'd be younger' and 'You wouldn't be able to handle it, you're too old' and 'We're looking for young, fresh-out-of-uni types'.

Our ovaries stop working and our skin starts to pleat; we're obsolete, invisible, embarrassing — and now we're unemployable too (unless you're a US politician or a justice of their Supreme Court, etc., but I'm guessing you're not).

Dr Jen Gunter, author of *The Menopause Manifesto*, says that as they age men get distinguished and women get diminished. While men are the silver foxes, we women are either cougars or nannas, mutton dressed as lamb or letting ourselves go. We're used to that, of course. We've been through years of being deemed either so thin it looks unhealthy or getting a bit porky. Everyone has an opinion about what we should look like. When I arrived in my thirties, several people said it was time to cut my hair into a bob because I was too old to be wearing it long now. At what seems the glorious height of my youth, I was meant to start ageing gracefully.

There are definite rules, and there is judgement for women who choose to break them. When Ari Seth Cohen (the US photographer with the fabulous *Advanced Style* blog that showcases über-stylish older people) posted a shot of a mature woman baring her midriff he had comments from people who were shocked and disgusted. 'Let's rid ourselves of antiquated and ageist standards of beauty and allow everyone to be who they want be,' pleaded Ari on his Facebook page.

It's time we looked at any and all ageist attitudes with horror and shame, just as we (hopefully) do homophobia and racism. I don't demand a special level of respect because I'm older and I don't claim to be any wiser or better. I'd just like to be treated the way I was 30 years ago: be visible and valuable, not diminished by age, not looked down on by people who haven't got to this point yet. I don't want to lose my currency just because I've gained a bigger back story.

And that's why OK Boomer is not OK.

~

Laila Harré

'Things are great now in so many ways.'

Former member of parliament Laila Harré experienced her first hot flush at the age of 43 when she was standing on the starting line of a half-marathon. 'It was a cold, miserable morning and I felt my whole body sort of heat up,' she recalls. 'At first I thought there was something wrong with me. From there I guess I started having the odd menopausal symptom.'

Now in her mid-fifties, Laila is through the transition. She is about to take on a new work challenge and recently became a grandmother. But there has been a journey to get where she is today.

In 2009 Laila was diagnosed with breast cancer and had a double mastectomy. Although she wasn't taking any oestrogen-blocking medication, the heat surges picked up from then on, and there were a few years where she was experiencing 20 or 30 flushes a day.

'The people I worked with over that time just got used to me turning the temperature up or down, putting clothes on and taking them off. I was very open about what was happening,' she says.

Looking back, there were things she should have done more about. 'The biggest one was my sex drive. I dried up and found sex painful. Fortunately, in my post-menopause life this has been completely resolved, which is fantastic.'

Laila's moods were also affected. At various

times in her life she has suffered from anxiety; now she felt really low and chose to take anti-depressants for the first time.

A couple of years ago all of those symptoms eased. 'Things are really great now in so many ways,' says Laila. 'I've been off anti-depressants for some time, I don't have the same mood issues, my anxiety is much more managed.'

She is a calmer person than she was in her younger years when she had much more to prove. 'My impatience levels have dropped substantially and my acceptance levels have risen. Over the past few years my work has been mainly coaching younger people, and I feel like my ability to do that is way better than it would have been ten years ago.'

Evenness of mood is just one bonus of life post-menopause. There is also a refreshingly changed attitude towards sex with her partner of 36 years.

'When you're menstruating and in a relationship, sex is so tied up with having children or not having children, preventing them or getting them,' says Laila. 'So I've found it really liberating to be able to dissociate my sexuality from my fertility, and instead be able to think: do I want it?'

'Age has changed and the fifties are still young . . . There used to be this idea that the minute a woman hit 40 she was a goner, she became completely invisible and was meant to act like she was on the brink of death.'

— novelist Marian Keyes, *The Shift* podcast

Chapter 15
Re-invention: getting ready for the second act

At first I struggled with getting older. I found it weird that men weren't gawking, beeping their horns, or whistling for me to come over. I didn't realise how much my self-esteem was dependent on the adoration of others. Now I recognise it. Now I know what bullshit that is/was. Now I know I didn't need that anymore. Now I'm free. We don't become obsolete if no one is looking. We don't disappear if others don't find us attractive. Now we know we don't need others' validation or approval. Now we are free. @stylemesunday

US fashion blogger and stylist Natalie Lee — aka *stylemesunday* — kindly gave me permission to use this Instagram post of hers, which I loved because it sums up what's so great about midlife. The male gaze has lost its intensity, and that is liberating. We get to be ourselves *for ourselves*. It's re-invention time.

For some that is going to be exciting, but for others it will be daunting. I found it difficult enough to invent myself the first time around. Do I really have to do it again?

My sister-in-law Diana went through a phase of giving me these kaftan/mumu-type garments she had bought while travelling the world. They were spacious and welcoming. I was certain that I could expand to almost any size at all and they would continue to accommodate me. And the comfort; it was insane. So long as I avoided my reflection in the mirror, there was really no down-side to them.

The mumus went to the op shop (sorry, Diana), as I didn't want to re-invent myself as the woman who wore them. Since then I've struggled to redefine my sense of style. Who do I want to be, and what do I want to look like? Those seem to be two questions that are tied together.

I don't know if you've ever come across the Red Hat Society? This is a worldwide movement and you have to be over 50 to join up. It was inspired by a 1992 poem called 'Warning' by the late Jenny Joseph, which starts:

Re-invention: getting ready for the second act

When I am an old woman I shall wear purple
With a red hat which doesn't go, and doesn't suit me.

Join the Red Hat Society, and the deal is that you dress in a red hat and purple coat combo, go on outings and have a lot of fun. A battalion of them, en masse, is quite a sight. However, while I applaud the sentiment, and fully approve of going out and having fun, I think they've rather misinterpreted the poem, which goes on to detail all the many ways Jenny Joseph planned to misbehave, like spending her pension on brandy and satin sandals. She wasn't suggesting that we rip our way out of our old skin, roaring and crying, just to turn into carbon copies of each other! She was saying that this was our chance to be impractical, wild, eccentric and badly behaved, if that's what we wanted — but most of all to be the selves we always wanted to be.

It's not only the red hat ladies who are carbon copies. A few years back I'd been taking part in an event at the Auckland Writers Festival and had arranged to meet a good friend afterwards in the foyer. She has cropped grey hair and is stylish in a practical way. I stepped through the door from backstage, looked about, and at least three-quarters of the women there fitted that exact description. It was very difficult to track my particular one down. Afterwards I wondered what on earth was happening. Were we all destined to morph into the same person? Is it welcome to clone-dom rather than welcome to crone-dom?

During my tireless research (i.e. wasting time on social media) I came across Emma John on Instagram. Actually I'd already come across Emma years ago when we ended up on the same trip to Shanghai. She's got one of those warm, vibrant personalities and I was determined to make her be my friend, but somehow she got away on me. So I was intrigued to discover that in midlife Emma has re-invented herself as a wardrobe consultant under the name Sisterhood of Style. She promises to help her clients unlock their sense of style and promises they'll never again ask the question 'What am I going to wear?' Emma will work with the clothes they have, take them shopping for new ones, or style them for a special event. And while she doesn't cater exclusively for midlife women, it is where there's a lot of need for her services.

Emma went through a surgically induced menopause in her forties and says she experienced an eighteen-month period where her body, mental health and personality changed completely. She was depressed, felt hopeless, tired and unmotivated, and cried at the drop of a hat. She put on weight, and was dizzy and itchy. There were a lot of symptoms and HRT was a lifesaver. Within a week she felt a change for the better.

When Emma started talking about midlife and menopause in her Instagram videos, she got a huge response. Some people aren't interested in joining the conversation, but a lot have been pleased to hear her saying things they've been thinking and feeling.

Her style is definitely not mine. She is maximalist — or 'extra' as I think we're meant to call it now. When she puts together an outfit for herself, it often involves more than one bright colour and several accessories, and she is definitely not invisible! But I do like her philosophy of clothes — as an extra layer of confidence — and I love the way she is empowering women.

Q&A with Emma John of Sisterhood of Style

Who are your clients and what are they telling you?
I specialise in midlife, menopause and motherhood, because these are three of the biggest changes we experience and often they can be the catalyst for an overhaul or life change. What women who've hit menopause often tell me is that they've put on weight, they've lost interest in clothes, it's all too hard — help! Many have lost confidence in themselves, and what used to work for them doesn't anymore so they don't believe they can put an outfit together that looks great.

Has your own style changed in midlife?

I think I've found my style, which is maximalist chic with a hint of head librarian on acid! I adore colour and, in fact, I'm better in colour. While I feel very strong in black, often I can't wear it anymore because I don't feel like me. Mostly, though, I think what I've accepted is that I wear the size of clothes that suit me and the size that fits me.

How do you approach working with clients?

I want them to feel good, to have excitement around going shopping again and enjoy opening up their wardrobe and putting outfits together. I'll always stress that I'm not there to make them look like me. But I will try to change their mindset and help them realise they can stand out and feel fantastic. Often I'll talk about clothes being external armour, helping you through the day.

Confidence comes down to three things for me. The first is being comfortable. No pulling, pushing, tying, untying, pulling your bra strap up, not having to shift the outfit once it's on. The second is not caring what others think — so dressing for yourself. Whether it's all in black or bright colour, the person you're trying to impress is *you*. And finally I think there's an energy that clothes can give you if you allow them to. There's a little bit of work to be done in terms of effort, but if you're feeling good in your outfit, you do feel better; you walk into a room more confidently, you feel more positive, and that energy is contagious.

I hope that after they've worked with me, clients will at least have the confidence to put together an outfit that makes them feel good and can be the suit of armour they need to walk out the door.

Magazine stories about midlife and beyond tend to be illustrated with photos of attractive grey-haired couples, skin glowing, heads thrown back and laughing gaily as they stride down a beach together or cycle through the countryside. They are fake people. If they are the only inspirational role models apart from the ageless women like Nicole Kidman and J.Lo (I've heard them described as 'the perennials'), then we need better role models, because they're not very real either.

I don't enjoy change and the prospect of re-inventing my outer layer isn't exciting me. I keep buying the wrong thing. My attempt to embrace colour resulted in a collection of orange bangles that mostly live in a drawer. The floaty cover-ups I thought would become outfit staples look like they belong to some other woman. I'm never going to wow like Emma John, who turned up for coffee in a dazzling bright-yellow skirt. Or Peta Mathias and the glorious divas of *Advanced Style*, much as I admire their flamboyance.

There are other ways to re-invent yourself, of course. Midlife seems the ideal time to strike out and try new things. By now you should be pretty damn good at whatever it is you've been doing for all these years, so why not see how else those skills can be applied? This is going to look different for everybody. It might mean a job change, exploring creativity, taking up a new sport, doing more learning, or returning to something you once loved but put aside in the busy-ness of juggling family and career.

If you are considering a change, there is a really cool Japanese concept I've just come across called *ikigai*. This loosely translates as 'reason for being' and is often illustrated with a Venn diagram with four overlapping qualities — what you love, what you are good at, what the world needs and what you can be paid for. Where you are in life will dictate which of these you prioritise. For some financial security will be uppermost, for others fulfilment more important — but you should always start with what you are good at. (There are lots of examples of the Venn diagram to be found with a quick google.)

About a decade ago, another journalist cheerfully said to me: 'We've had our careers, haven't we? The younger ones are coming through now and they're so talented.' At the time I was shocked, because, no, I didn't feel like I'd had my career. There were still many things I wanted to achieve, and in a way it felt like I was only just beginning.

With respect to young people who indeed are talented, I still feel much the same. There is a lot left for me to do. Hopefully this is the middle of my adult life, not the end, and I'm saying yes to opportunities. Like writing this book, for instance. Or making my first podcast, *Book Bubble*, with fellow author Stacy Gregg during the first national lockdown. Or taking a ten-week online screen-writing course, which was challenging but really got my brain firing.

I'd like to do more learning. A permaculture course maybe. Or pottery classes (I think it's the law that you have to take those at the moment). I'd like to ride a decent dressage test. Do a Great Walk. Write a TV drama series or a psychological thriller. Get better at speaking Italian. Learn te reo Māori.

Always contrary, I'd also like to learn to live more slowly.

My hormones might have changed, but that hasn't rendered me obsolete or incapable. At this point nothing is over except the ability to make babies and the need to have tampons stashed everywhere I go. And Emma John is right: I am still allowed to stand out and feel fabulous. Maybe I'll try actually wearing those orange bangles. Who knows what I'll do after that? Who knows what you'll do? All that possibility just waiting for us — it's quite exciting.

We can no longer create life . . . so now it's time to create our own lives.

Sarah-Kate Lynch

'You can't listen to the voice inside your head if it's saying you're over the hill.'

For years Sarah-Kate Lynch wrote novels, but then in her fifties she pivoted (before pivoting was even a thing!) and carved out a whole new career writing television drama. She is a good friend and it has been interesting to watch how much hard work and dedication she has put into re-inventing herself. Happily it's paid off and the psychological thriller series she created, *The Sounds*, has been a hit on international streaming channels.

Menopause snuck up pretty quietly on Sarah-Kate. 'I didn't have any hot flushes,' she says. 'And because I'd had a partial hysterectomy my periods had stopped ages before. It's only recently, looking back, that I've realised in my early fifties my self-confidence suffered. That was a time when I should have been confident in my work history and my instinct, but I was second-guessing myself constantly in a slightly anxious way. Maybe it wasn't anything to do with menopause, although my GP did say something funny to me at that time — she said, "If anything shit is happening it's menopause." '

Sarah-Kate's faltering self-confidence coincided with the Global Financial Crisis and a downturn in book sales. She had to do something else, but what? Realising that TV drama was having a golden age, she approached Kelly Martin, the chief executive of production company South Pacific Pictures, and asked if she could sit in with the storyliners working on *Shortland Street* and see how it was done.

So suddenly she found herself the oldest and most inexperienced person in a room full of other people who knew exactly what they were doing. It was tough, she admits.

'But I wasn't going to let my inner voice tell me I shouldn't be there. You've got to grit your teeth and get past that feeling of OMG OMG! I think when you're going to make a shift in your fifties you have to give yourself the credit of having something to bring to the table, even if it's not the exact thing that the table wants!'

At least in your fifties you've got life experience and have developed a few instincts worth trusting. Armed with those things and an impressive work ethic — reading books, doing online study, listening to podcasts, and being mentored by other writers — Sarah-Kate located her missing self-confidence eventually.

In a creative business, she never takes success

for granted. 'But I've got more ideas at this stage of my life, and in a strange way I've got more energy than before,' she says. 'So you can't listen to the voice inside your head if it's saying you're over the hill or it's a young person's game. You can't listen to any of that.'

'There's always a frightening point, when your face starts to change — and it lasts quite a long time, maybe ten years — then you find actually that you've grown into an older face.'

— *Charlotte Rampling in* The Independent

Chapter 16

Exercise to energise, not exhaust

If you google the words 'exercise, menopause, midlife', what you'll find is a whole lot of websites offering the advice that you should exercise more, much more. Lift heavier weights, increase your heart rate, up the intensity, exercise harder, longer, faster. The assumption is that you're a middle-aged woman so you're probably struggling to get off the sofa. But quite possibly you are already doing a lot of high-intensity exercise and it isn't feeling as good as it used to.

The current generation of middle-aged women grew up with gym culture. We had the leg warmers for our Jane Fonda workouts in the 1980s. We did a ten-minute sweat with Richard Simmons. We tried step aerobics, high-impact, low-impact, bodypump, combat and jam, Jazzercise, Zumba. Some of us ran marathons or did triathlons (not me).

Many women have never slowed the pace. These days they're trying CrossFit or F45, they're doing ocean swims and cycling round Taupō. Injuries tend to happen more often than they used to, muscles take longer to recover, and many women, despite healthy eating and all that activity, are still struggling not to gain weight.

When I first came across the idea that in midlife highly active women might find that they need to exercise *less*, I thought it was a bit of a con. Then I talked to Wendy Sweet, and things started to make sense. Wānaka-based Wendy is a former nurse and personal trainer who re-invented herself in midlife, becoming a women's health and ageing educator. She studied for a PhD in Health, Sport and Human Performance at the University of Waikato, where she has also lectured in the Faculty of Health. And she created My Menopause Transformation, an international online programme with lifestyle changes that women use alongside, or instead of, HRT to support themselves through the midlife transition.

Wendy is very interested in reducing inflammation by eating well, managing stress and staying active *in an appropriate way* for your age and stage. She says that exercise should energise you, not exhaust you. Yes you need balance, strength and flexibility, yes you need cardio fitness, but you don't need to be pushing yourself in a programme that has been designed for a high-performance male.

There has been a lot of focus on younger female athletes who exercise intensely and don't consume enough calories, adversely affecting their hormones and bone density as a result (it's known as the female athlete triad). Midlife women seem to have been overlooked, however. No one is thinking too much about anything except the fact that exercise is good for *us* because it builds bone, is vital for cardiovascular health and can prevent weight gain. Hence the 'do more' message that we've got used to hearing, rather than specifically tailoring workouts to us.

Wendy describes having a light-bulb moment when she realised that most of the research around sport and exercise science has been conducted with men, younger people or Boomers over the age of 65. There is a gap in the knowledge, and midlife women are falling right into it. We're losing oestrogen, our joints and muscles hurt, we're hot, not sleeping and exhausted, and yet we're trying to push just as hard when we're exercising.

Speaking to women who were doing a lot of high-intensity exercise, Wendy heard over and over that it wasn't going well for them. Their bodies hurt more, their hot flushes were worse, and many were still putting on weight. This reflected her own experience of being a long-time fitness advocate who in middle age, still exercising and eating the way she always had, found herself gaining 15 kilos, struggling to sleep and feeling sore.

Wendy now believes that this is all a part of the female athlete triad, just at a different life stage; a time when our muscles are ageing and changing, and very intense exercise on a daily basis isn't necessarily the best thing for our bodies.

She isn't suggesting that anyone stops being active. But if you're exhausted and not sleeping, if life is super-busy and you're feeling overwhelmed, if your menopause symptoms are severe, then it's a sign that you may need to pull back on physical activity, at least for a while. Rather than lifting very heavy weights, you might be better off for a time with body resistance exercises like Pilates, which will also build core strength, flexibility and balance. Or taking a brisk walk in nature rather than pounding kilometres of concrete pavements at a run. While you need to keep moving, quite possibly you don't need to be swinging from ropes in a CrossFit session.

An exercise prescription for women as they age is only just emerging, especially in the area of heart health. And Wendy argues that a lot of this information isn't getting to women because it is rarely taught to health professionals. Also, the difference between 'exercise for healthy ageing' and 'exercise for performance' is often not recognised within the gym environment.

The perfect amount of exercise for you depends on your level of fitness, how busy you are, how well you sleep, how exhausted you feel, how active or sedentary your job is, and how much your muscles ache. That's true at any stage of life, but at this point get the balance wrong and you'll start to feel it more, especially with your menopause symptoms.

In her sixties now, Wendy is a very good advertisement for getting the exercise balance right.

Q&A with Wendy Sweet from My Menopause Transformation

Why is 'exercise to energise but not exhaust' the best fitness philosophy for midlife women?

The fitness industry has done a very good job of convincing women that they need to exercise intensely to lose weight. We're the first generation to come through with that belief system. If women are putting on weight even though they're exercising furiously, it's because they're not looking at the whole context. They might be busy all day, have a lot of stress in their home environment, be caring for their parents and also kids, working in quite physical jobs, or they may have more than one job which has a huge impact on their stress levels. A lot of them are arriving in menopause exhausted, so first they've got to unravel the inflammation that's been building up. Actually the very first thing they need to do is sleep all night, and they can't do that if they're over-training. I've had thousands of women on my programmes where I've said, we're pulling you back, we're going low and we'll do that until you're sleeping all night. It can take six months for these women to get there.

What sort of exercise do you do yourself?
Aerobic exercise and bodyweight exercise, rather than heavy weights, which will increase inflammation and cortisol and put your blood pressure up. That's the pathway I've followed. I also love to ski.

Over-exercising may not be your problem. You might be struggling to find the time or energy to do much activity at all. In midlife, some women will stop exercising altogether. Feeling burnt-out or unable to manage what they did before, they become discouraged and give up. Since this coincides with the natural weakening of bones and the stiffening of arteries and the swinging of moods, it adds up to poorer health overall.

The trouble for many of us is that we don't get to move enough in the course of our everyday lives. That might be due to desk-bound jobs, or simply because of the way the modern world has been designed. With our labour-saving devices, our screens and our cars, we've created what has been called a pandemic of physical inactivity.

I've spent a lot of time at my desk, moving only my fingers, while writing this book. Once I might have needed to get up and send a fax, or chat to a colleague; now it's easy not to move at all for hours on end. I don't feel good mentally or physically after too long at my laptop. And yet I have deadlines, and so that's what I keep doing.

Humans are meant to move. We evolved as hunter-gatherers covering 9–14 kilometres a day to find our food. Being too sedentary is bad for our health in a dizzying array of ways. Resting muscles produce fewer of the proteins that break down triglycerides — a type of fat found in the blood that is released for energy. And the absence of muscle contraction isn't helpful for the correct processing of blood glucose, either. One large US study found that sitting around for more than six hours a day makes you more likely to acquire a long list of conditions ranging from Alzheimer's to type 2 diabetes, cardiovascular problems and cancer, plus it raises the risk of an early death by 19%.[1]

There are solutions — sit/stand desks, walking meetings, Swiss balls, phones and watches that sound an alarm reminding us to get up and move around every 30 minutes. But many of us are still sitting for too long. One in eight New Zealand adults is active for less than half an hour a week.

One solution seems to be so-called 'exercise snacking' — small bursts of activity throughout a day to break up sedentary time. Even the first minute of exercise improves your health, just getting out of a chair and walking a few steps. So, climb the stairs instead of taking the lift. Bike to work. Go for a stroll at lunchtime rather than eating at your desk. Or just stand up and have a walk around the office every 30 minutes — that all counts as activity. It's ideal to get in a longer stint of daily exercise, too, but if time is short then micro-bouts are better than nothing at all.

Perhaps one of the most compelling reasons to keep moving in midlife is that exercise has been shown to have a positive effect on brain metabolism, delaying cognitive decline. It increases the size of the hippocampus, the part of the brain that controls short-term memory. A Swedish study concluded that women with high cardiovascular fitness in middle age are nearly 90% less likely to develop dementia decades later compared with women who are only moderately fit.[2] But even ten minutes of gentle exercise is enough to improve memory function.

Staying active slows the ageing process in other ways,

keeping the muscles and cardiovascular system biologically decades younger. I interviewed a scientist called Scott Trappe, the director of the Human Performance Laboratory at Ball State University in Indiana, who told me that between the ages of 70 and 80 is when the major decline starts to happen. The septuagenarian runners who took part in his team's study[3] had the heart and lung capacities, and muscle fitness, of healthy people in their early forties. Many had switched to cycling after their knees packed in, but they loved to exercise and weren't giving it up.

Scott told me that one of the advantages of having a bigger cardiovascular engine is it means a person has a greater reserve, meaning they can rebound more success-fully from adverse life events such as periods of illness.

'There's a sort of aerobic frailty threshold,' he explained. 'The data is pretty clear that when you dip below this threshold that's the big transition between independence and dependence. Once you're at those very low thresholds, it's really difficult to get back above them. So that's a game-changer and it's why having a reserve is key.'

Scott said a mix of aerobic and strength training is ideal, but the most important thing is that you enjoy whatever you do enough to want to work out for at least 30–45 minutes a day.

'There is no one formula that is perfect for everyone,' he told me. 'Some are more into running, some cycling, weight training, walking, yoga, or whatever. All these things are beneficial so long as you're consistent. At the end of the day, exercise wins. It has so many positive systemic benefits. Even when you get into your eighties you still benefit, although those benefits aren't as robust as when you're young.'

~

So during your 8–10 years of menopause transition you might want to take things down a couple of gears and go more gently. Extreme exercise might not be the best idea at this age and stage. But definitely don't give up altogether is the message that all this research is telling us. Keep moving and often, even if it's not all that far.

5 exercise snacks

1. Hopping on one leg for two minutes a day can strengthen hip bones in post-menopausal women, according to researchers at the UK's Loughborough University.[4]
2. Sit-to-stand — rise from an upright seated position on a chair, and then return to the seated position. Keep your arms folded across your chest to avoid using them to help. See how

many sit-to-stands you can perform in 1 minute.

3. Calf raises — Start with your feet flat on the floor and rise up on to your tip-toes as high as you can, then return to the starting position with feet flat on the floor. Complete as many as you can in 1 minute.

4. If you have a stationary bike or rowing machine, just jump on that for a minute or so.

5. Stand up and jog on the spot for 20 seconds. Or do 20 seconds of squats or push-ups.

Selina Tusitala Marsh

'You can't stay the same out of fear.'

I have a girl-crush on the poet Selina Tusitala Marsh. She is beautiful, with the best hair ever, as well as thoughtful and smart. I interviewed her years ago when she launched her first poetry collection *Fast Talking PI*, and her career has gone from strength to strength since then.

In midlife Selina made a creative change, writing and illustrating children's books — beginning with the award-winning graphic memoir *Mophead* — and there have been changes for her personally, too.

When I catch up with her she is about to turn 50 and not entirely sure what that's supposed to look like.

'But I'm not interested in what other people think I should be looking like or behaving like,' she says, with certainty. 'And I'm not taking on board anything negative about it.'

She celebrated her forty-ninth birthday by getting her hands tattooed with the traditional Samoan tuālima, and says it felt like an initiation into a new facet of Selina. 'It marked a beautiful transition.'

At this point in her life she has given herself permission to no longer need permission. For a Pasifika woman who feels an obligation to serve her community, it's a big deal to live on her own terms, do the things that give her energy and fulfilment, and say no to the rest.

'I'm cultivating really meaningful relationships, the ones I want to cultivate, not the ones I feel obligated to,' she explains.

Selina describes this time as 'a new season', and it is one that has changed her in many ways. It has seen her relocate from her long-time home on Waiheke Island to an inner-city sky-scraping apartment. It has taken her on an epic road trip that was meant to last a week but ended up as two months of travel around New Zealand, living out of a suitcase and staying with friends and family. And she has whittled down her personal belongings after reading about Courtney Carver's minimalist fashion challenge Project 333 and realising that owning less brings mental clarity.

'I thought: who am I waiting for to come and design my life the way I want it? If not me, then who?' says Selina. 'You can't stay the same out of fear.'

With her children grown up, this is a time of freedom and she is valuing the chance to live in a way she never could when she was younger.

'I lived my twenties quite responsibly,' Selina explains. 'Samoans tend to be at home, then get married. We don't go out and explore the world on our own.'

She isn't sure what the future holds and describes her life as like being in a maze, following Ariadne's threads, taking the next step and the next, and being okay with detours that her younger self wouldn't have had time for. Most of all she is leaning into change, even if sometimes that might make things more difficult.

'I don't particularly like doing difficult things, but I've just proven that I can,' she says. 'And I can come out the other end and flourish.'

'The freedom that comes with no longer being fertile is huge.'

— Cynthia Nixon, Stella *magazine*

Chapter 17

Some thoughts on men

Men? We do all the things and once a fortnight they push a lawnmower around. They think their jobs are more important than ours, get paid more for doing them and expect to be congratulated in three languages if they take the bins out. (If this isn't your arrangement then congratulations, but I suspect it's the reality for many midlife women.)

Do we *really* need to worry about how men are coping with our menopause? I didn't think so. In fact, I wasn't going to write this chapter at all. But we can't ignore men. They're here, there and everywhere, all around us.

Men aren't one great homogenous mass. There are men

who really don't want to know about your menopause, and if you mention it they'll look like you're trying to give them the score for a rugby game they haven't yet watched. There are men who are jovially embarrassed about your flushed, sweaty moments. There are men who blame everything *they* don't like on *your* time of life. Men who assume you are going mad and there's nothing to be done about it. And men who are forensically interested in exactly what is going on with you, because they really want to understand. Any and all of these reactions could be wrong, depending on a woman's mood at any given time. That's probably not men's fault.

Still, if our menopause is a difficult time for them to navigate, then their man-opause isn't easy for us either. Outwards signs of this include grumpiness, mansplaining and ranting, then more grumpiness when you point out they're doing those things. There may also be a reluctance to try anything new and suddenly starting to say things like 'that's not my cup of tea'. Finger-wagging other motorists while driving. Not listening to a thing you say, then claiming you never tell them anything. Their six-pack turning into a keg. Moobs. Less energy. Low motivation. Difficulty sleeping, loss of muscle mass, fatigue and, last but definitely not least, erectile dysfunction.

Whether the man-opause — or the andropause — is actually a thing is up for debate. Testosterone levels in men do drop, but in a gradual way, at less than 2% a year from midlife onwards, and many older men still have levels in the normal range.

Impotence has tended to be the aspect of being an ageing male that gets the most attention and, just as with women, there have been many attempts over the years to find a remedy. In the 1800s physiologist Charles-Édouard Brown-Séquard injected himself with a rejuvenating elixir made from the extracts of animal testes that he claimed gave him greater vigour and 'increased the arc of his urine'. Testicular extract became a popular therapy for a while, as did the terrifying-sounding testicular tissue grafts from baboons and monkeys. Unsurprisingly, neither treatment caught on over the longer term.

Today, testosterone treatment is advised only for men with abnormally low levels of the hormone — or 'low-T' as it's known — if they are experiencing symptoms and blood tests confirm that there is a problem. It can improve mood, energy, libido and body composition in men who really need it. But there are side-effects, including an increase in prostate size and decreased sperm production, and older men on TRT (testosterone replacement therapy) could face higher cardiac risks.

And so men with mildly lowered levels are encouraged to try to boost their testosterone naturally by losing weight if necessary, drinking less alcohol, reducing stress, staying active and getting enough sleep.

Man-opause or not, if your male partner is more

grumpy and you're more 'ragey', then things are going to get fraught. Relationships can get broken in midlife. The median age at divorce is 47 for men and 44 for women, according to Statistics New Zealand.[1]

Not every woman is with a man. The lesbians I spoke to laughed wryly when I asked them about going through menopause together. They said that sharing PMT prepares you for the oncoming storm, but it's helpful to be with a partner who's a generation younger or older so that you're not totally in sync once menopause hits. On the whole they didn't think they had it any easier, although they felt more understood.

~

I found that all relationships were more difficult at my peri-menopausal heights. There were people I saw a lot less of out of fear I might tell them what I really thought. I'm sure I was more difficult to live with, but I was all out of sympathy and really didn't care.

Menopause should be taught to school-girls and boys in biology lessons. I don't remember it ever being mentioned back in the dark ages when I was being educated at a girls' school, although they showed us a very graphic film about the birth of a baby and we were given a small photograph of a penis with the words 'not actual size' printed next to it (shortly afterwards, I was ejected from the class for giggling). If kids knew more about it from the start, then they might not be so unprepared when it actually happens to them or their mothers and partners.

Men I spoke to seemed confused by the way their female partners were changing. They talked of 'walking on eggshells', and of parking the car outside the house but not wanting to go in because they didn't know which version of the person they loved was going to greet them. Men didn't understand why sex had changed — their partners were less interested, or wanted the light out, or didn't want to dress up in that sexy corset anymore (because they didn't feel as sexy in it). Men seemed utterly disoriented. Several made jokes about it at first, but then it became clear that they felt hurt and rejected; lots were trying to be supportive and weren't sure how; and there were men who said that their partners didn't want to talk about it. Men wanted help but didn't know where to turn.

If we want our relationships to survive, then we do have to consider how our menopause is affecting our partner — whatever gender that partner happens to be. I think life in general would be improved if we were all a little better at walking in other people's shoes. And to do so there needs to be a lot more understanding.

That means dropping the M-bomb into conversation. Mentioning hot flushes when you're having them. When your partner asks 'What's wrong', actually telling them. Admitting it if that new flesh duvet wrapped around your middle is making you feel less than fabulous. Talking about that emotional roller-coaster you're on. Asking them to do more than their share for a bit because you're exhausted and not coping.

If your partner doesn't want to listen, then talk a lot louder.

~

Kate Rodger

'I felt like I was scarring my children's lives.'

In her regular slot on TV3's *The AM Show*, entertainment editor Kate Rodger usually talks about celebrities and movies. In August 2021 she did something very different, opening up to host Ryan Bridge about her menopause experience. She told him about the hot flushes, the mood swings, the brain fog — for New Zealand television this was a milestone moment.

For Kate, although she was ready to discuss all that, it was an emotional experience. 'When I came off-air I burst into tears, which I didn't expect,' she says. 'And then my phone went absolutely crazy.'

I caught up with her a few days later when she was still struggling to respond to all the messages that had flooded in from women who wanted to share their menopause experiences with her. The segment was still getting thousands of views online, with only a few comments from men who didn't want to hear about women's bits over their breakfast.

Like so many of us, Kate missed the signs of peri-menopause. In her case, having a baby at the age of 45 probably meant she was too busy to notice until it got really obvious that something was changing.

'I had instant weight gain around my middle,' she recalls. 'Suddenly I didn't fit things and that annoyed the hell out of me. I lost the elasticity in my face pretty much overnight.'

Kate was being woken six or seven times a night by hot flushes. She started having dizzy spells that literally put her on her knees on the kitchen floor. But it was the mood swings that shocked her most.

'I felt like I was scarring my children's lives,' she says. 'I'd pull up into the carport in a happy mood, thinking I couldn't wait to see them, and then I'd walk in and within a breath I'd be postal. I couldn't control the outbursts of rage. My moods affected the mood of the whole house and this went on for months and months.'

After weighing up the pros and cons, she decided to take HRT. Kate would prefer not to take medication, and one factor to consider was that her mother had had breast cancer. But that risk is balanced by the fact that Kate rarely drinks alcohol these days. And most importantly, the treatment has brought relief from her symptoms.

'The weird thing about putting oestrogen into my body is it feels like eating carrots and celery every day,' she says, 'It's like this miracle hormone that does everything. So I'm not ready to let it go quite yet.'

Kate is on a mission now, talking about menopause not only on-air but also to the younger women she works with, so they don't suddenly wake up to what is going on when they're three years into it.

'Knowledge is power,' she says. 'There are so many lifestyle choices you can make leading up to peri-menopause that might make a difference.'

Chapter 18

Inflammation, telomeres and the science of ageing well

The word 'anti-ageing', which gets plastered all over pots and tubes of face cream, is obviously a nonsense. Nothing will prevent you ageing except premature death. So obviously none of us is anti ageing — what we want is to age well.

The elderly men and women I admire have a lot going on. They've got purpose and they push themselves. Those are the people I want to be when I get old, if at all possible. They are who I am re-inventing myself into.

Some things are out of my control. I can't do anything about the amount of vodka I drank in my twenties in that basement bar in London's Soho. Or the sun damage I acquired driving a convertible car in my forties. All I can influence is my behaviour now. And to age well from here onwards, all the evidence suggests that I need to keep a lid on inflammation.

~

Inflammation isn't wholly bad. When it's operating properly it is the body's natural protective response. If you hurt yourself, white blood cells flood the area to deal with any foreign particles, and platelets rush in to stem the flow of blood. You might experience this as redness, swelling or pain, and that's quite normal.

The problem is that as our cells get older they become less efficient at turning off inflammation when it's done its job. The shrinking of our brains, the failing of our hearts, diabetes and cancer, our stiffer, frailer bodies — all are associated with this process. Its role in the ageing process has led to the coining of a word — inflammaging.

There is an increasing amount of evidence to show that our modern lifestyles may worsen this chronic systemic inflammation. What we eat and drink definitely has a role to play. Thinking of pulling the tab on a nice cold can of cola? Research from Mexico has linked consumption of fizzy drinks with a significant rise in levels of CRP (C-reactive protein), which is produced by the liver in response to inflammation — it was 50% higher in the otherwise healthy midlife women who drank the most soda.[1]

The ratio of omega-3 and omega-6 fatty acids in our diets has also been under scrutiny. We evolved eating equal amounts of both, but the Western diet has skewed to higher levels of the pro-inflammatory omega-6, largely because of widespread use of processed vegetable oils, and to lower levels of the anti-inflammatory omega-3, found in fish oil.

In 2014 epidemiologists from the University of South Carolina reviewed the available research around nutrition and inflammation, and produced the Dietary Inflammatory Index for use as a tool to assess various eating plans. It won't come as a huge surprise that, using this measure, fast-food diets have been shown to have strong pro-inflammatory potential. Sugar, trans fats, processed meats, fries and refined starchy carbs all rate as inflammatory. Excessive alcohol is definitely bad, as is too much sugar or salt.

Meanwhile the Mediterranean-style diet — rich in fresh vegetables, fruit, whole grains and fish — is anti-inflammatory, as are variations of it such as the MIND or DASH diets. The spice turmeric contains a compound called curcumin that has been shown to lower the levels of enzymes in the body that cause inflammation. Ginger has also been seen to influence inflammatory processes. Foods high in antioxidants and polyphenols, such as blueberries, apples, leafy greens, fatty fish, nuts, olive oil, tomatoes and green tea, are all touted as inflammation beaters. Coffee may have a friendly role, as may dark chocolate. And eating lots of nuts has consistently been shown to lower inflammation.

Diet is not the only lifestyle factor at play. Low physical fitness, poor oral hygiene, smoking and obesity are all linked to a higher degree of inflammation. Other pro-inflammatory factors include over-exercising, allergies that haven't been identified, infections people didn't know they had, exposure to mould toxins in older or leaky homes, and exposure to heavy metals and chemical toxins.

Prolonged stress acts at a cellular level and has lasting effects. When we're under stress, our central nervous system sends out signals to activate our immune cells. Those cells kick in with the inflammatory response that is part of our body's defence system. If the stress continues and there is an excessive inflammatory response, the body tries to adapt by shutting down the immune system and we become more susceptible to diseases and viruses.

Mindfulness, meditation techniques, yoga and tai chi dampen the activity of genes associated with inflammation. It seems that it doesn't matter which one you choose to take up, the result will be that your genes won't be activated as persistently to produce the signals that cause inflammation.

~

The other aspect of the biology of ageing that we can influence with our lifestyle is our telomeres. Often compared to the hard plastic tip on a shoelace, telomeres are structures of DNA at the end of our chromosomes. Every time a cell divides, its telomere shortens, until finally the cell is unable to divide any further and becomes what is called senescent. This can have serious consequences for your health. When you have too many senescent cells in your bloodstream, your immune system becomes compromised; too many in the walls of your blood vessels, and your arteries stiffen; too many in your skin, and it becomes thin, etc. Therefore the shorter your telomeres are, the higher your chance of dying of a chronic illness such as diabetes, heart disease and even some cancers.

Nobel-prize-winning molecular biologist Elizabeth Blackburn discovered how telomeres work while she was experimenting on pond scum. At her lab in the University of California she made an exciting discovery: in some conditions, the telomeres in pond scum actually grew longer. She saw the same thing happen in yeast cells and was intrigued. It turned out there was an enzyme at work — which Blackburn's lab named telomerase — that can maintain a telomere by building it back up each time a cell divides. Cells with enough telomerase appeared to maintain themselves indefinitely.

There are efforts to convert telomerase into an elixir of youth, but these are progressing very slowly because, as with any treatment that tinkers with the cells, researchers are walking a tightrope between slowing ageing and causing cancer. For the same reason you might want to take a cautious approach to any supplements that claim to activate telomerase. For now it's unknown territory, and a safer approach might be to control the lifestyle factors that influence telomere length without any attendant risk.

Long-lasting stress appears to a major factor in shortening them, as Elizabeth Blackburn's team found in a study involving mothers caring for children with chronic conditions.[2] Telomerase-boosting strategies that Elizabeth Blackburn suggests include meditation, mindfulness-based stress reduction and yoga, in particular Kirtan Kriya which involves chanting and the tapping of fingers. In a trial involving people caring for family members with dementia,[3] those who practised this for twelve minutes a day for two months increased telomerase levels by 43% and decreased gene expression related to inflammation. The Chinese moving meditation qigong has also been shown to increase telomerase levels.[4]

~

Not everyone agrees that behavioural factors are going to make changes on a cellular level that are significant enough to hold off the diseases of old age. But Elizabeth Blackburn seems convinced that it's worth a go. In 2017 she told UK newspaper *The Guardian* 'I exercise, but I don't spend hours at the gym; I have a good diet, but am not fanatical about food; and I try to think about the effect of stress. I practise micro-meditations which I think help.'

Live for long enough, and no matter how healthy your habits, your body will deteriorate to some degree. Science is trying to change that, with millions being spent by the biotech companies of Silicon Valley as they try to hack the code of lasting health and longevity. We may be on the cusp of treatments that slow down the cellular ageing of the body, meaning that we'll remain fitter, stronger, and less prone to aching hips and creaky knees. Other treatments like gene therapy and stem cell therapy may lie in the future.

Right now, though, all we can do is obey the usual rules of living well. They are the same things we hear over and over again, but they are especially important in the menopause transition, so I'll repeat them just in case.

- Eat a wholefood diet rich in vegetables and oily fish.
- Avoid sugar, saturated fat and too much salt.
- Don't smoke.
- Look after your teeth.
- Get vaccinated.
- Get enough sleep.
- Get enough-but-not-too-much exercise.

Don't Sweat it

- Limit chemical exposure.
- Wash your hands.
- Try not to breathe polluted air.
- Get outdoors into nature.
- Soak up enough vitamin D but not too many UV rays.
- Connect with other people.
- Use your brain.

'Menopause makes you feel fat, ugly and awful. You puff up, can't sleep and you're overheating all the time . . . But I feel better now.'

— *Hilary Barry*, New Zealand Woman's Weekly

Chapter 19

And so to sum up

The menopause revolution isn't about medicating every midlife woman. It's not about treating older women as if they are deficient in anything, including hormones. This revolution is about knowledge — learning it, airing it, sharing it.

I wasn't prepared for menopause — didn't know anything and tried not to think about it. As a younger woman, if I did any thinking at all then it was in terms of losing my fertility and perhaps getting the odd flush.

After being a health journalist for years, I thought I knew more about menopause. Still I knew next to nothing, even after I'd actually been through it. Now I'm shocked at how many fake facts I've found while navigating my way through the information that's out there. Mostly I'm shocked at the lack of agency women are being given over their bodies. *My doctor says I've got to come off HRT . . . I can't get my GP to prescribe it and got anti-depressants instead . . . No one told me there was a solution to my dry vagina . . . I don't want to take hormones so I thought the only alternative was to get on with things.* I heard all of these things, far too often, and I'd like to think that future generations of women in Aotearoa won't be saying them, too.

The menopause revolution is about empowering women to make their own choices. With more knowledge we will be freer. And doctors will be our trusted advisers, not our decision-makers or gatekeepers.

By 2025 there will be over a billion women around the world in menopause — that's 12% of the global population, a battalion of us, and according to the venture capital firm Female Founders Fund we represent a $US600 billion opportunity for industry. Currently we're under-served and asking for more. A survey by the organisation found that 78% of women said menopause had interfered with their lives to some degree, only 36% felt they had been prepared for it, and 71% said they would benefit from a community around the menopause experience.[1]

We are a tech-savvy generation, one that, by and large, has had more education and career opportunities than any women before, more control over our lives, more financial independence, more choice. Are we really going to suffer stigma and silence at this time of our lives? Are we going to allow menopause to remain a mystery? I don't think so.

Let's talk about it and normalise it. Let's spread the word so that younger women know what's coming and they can ask for help if they need it. Let's disrupt menopause, once and for all. A woman's life shouldn't be a journey towards irrelevance and invisibility. So let's disrupt ageism, too. The revolution is happening.

Since most of us are tech-savvy, a lot of this disruption is happening online where women are beginning to connect with each other and create the communities we need. In 2015 a Facebook group called What Would Virginia Woolf Do? was started for midlife women by an American called Nina Lorez Collins. The name was a dark joke — as in should we just wander into a river as the writer Virginia Woolf did? — and the answer, of course, was no. Stories and experiences were shared, the whole thing grew and grew, and now it's changed its name to Revel and continues to expand. There are events, podcasts, workshops, parties, sex chats — it's like a giant international club for women over 40, and its success is a clear sign that the menopausal billion want to talk about it.

Here in New Zealand the Menopause Over Martinis movement is gathering pace. It all started as a single pot-luck dinner hosted by a Wellington freelance writer called Sarah Connor. In her late forties Sarah was blindsided by a whole medley of menopause symptoms, including anxiety, panic attacks, insomnia and low mood. It took months for her to work out that what was happening was entirely normal, and the knowledge came as an immense relief.

Sarah started taking HRT, and once back on a more even keel it occurred to her that her friends must be going through the same thing — hence that first pot-luck dinner to discuss all things menopause.

'We talked about what we did and didn't know, we asked each other questions, and all kinds of stuff came up; it was just so much fun,' says Sarah.

More dinners followed. They were so successful that Sarah created a website, with tips for other women who wanted to host similar evenings. This has snowballed to the point where she is getting interest from overseas, Menopause Over Martinis gatherings are happening around the country, and in July 2021 there was the first mass meeting in Wellington with 60 guests and not a moment's silence.

Cocktails are not compulsory, but you are encouraged to stay on topic and a lot of 'aha moments' tend to happen around those dinner tables. Women realise what is going on, why it's going on and, most importantly, that they are not alone.

'Many women say the best thing is walking into a room full of people who are there to talk about peri-menopause and menopause,' says Sarah. 'It's an invitation to sit down and be really open. There are no barriers, no shame. When you give them permission to talk about it, people have so much to say.'

She recalls as a girl being presented with a booklet that detailed the changes she could expect to happen to her body in puberty. 'For menopause there's nothing,' she says. 'No brochure, no poster, no trip to your GP when you turn 40 — it's extraordinary.'

Having gone into her own peri-menopause unprepared and uninformed, Sarah is now doing her best to make sure other women get a better start on this life-stage. 'It isn't just a woman's issue,' she points out. 'It's an all-of-society issue. It affects our partners, our colleagues, our children.'

We're not the only ones on fire — the whole topic of menopause is blazing now. In September 2021, Ireland announced it would be establishing specialist menopause clinics across the country, beginning in Dublin. In the UK, where the menopause revolution is really rolling, the government has reduced prescription charges on HRT, is creating a menopause task force to drive change in workplace policy, medical school training, public health messaging and school curriculums, and has promised to make menopause a priority in an upcoming women's health strategy.

'If the menopause were an illness, or indeed a condition that impacted every man, it's unlikely that financial support would be so woeful, or public understanding so negligible. Women have suffered long enough — I am determined to change that,' MP Carolyn Harris has said.

Also in the UK, psychotherapist Diane Danzebrink has created the not-for-profit organisation Menopause Support and the #MakeMenopauseMatter campaign to shatter the silence and improve support for midlife women. One of the things she has been calling for since 2015 is mandatory menopause education for all GPs. Recently her organisation surveyed the UK's 33 medical schools and found that 41% of them didn't have menopause education on the curriculum, effectively meaning that many doctors were leaving university with no training in it at all.

Eventually there won't only be better training, but also better treatments. There is excitement about a class of anti-psychotic drug, called NK3R antagonists, providing a non-hormonal way to control hot flushes by working to disrupt the signalling pathway. Clinical trials have been encouraging and it could be a game-changer for women who are unable to take hormones.

'Women deserve better' is the phrase that campaigners like Diane Danzebrink keep repeating, and they are starting to make a real difference. Progress must seem frustratingly slow at times, but hopefully it will mean that the next wave of women to enter peri-menopause will find themselves better served in every way.

~

As I put the finishing touches to this book it was World Menopause Month, October 2021, and it felt as if we had reached a tipping point, at least in terms of visibility.

Sophie, Countess of Wessex became the first member of Britain's royal family to talk about brain fog and other symptoms. 'You suddenly can't remember what on earth it was you were talking about. Try being on an engagement when that happens,' she said. 'Your words just go. And you're standing there going, "Hang on, I thought I was a reasonably intelligent person. What has just happened to me?" It's like someone has just gone and taken your brain out for however long before they pop it back in again, and you try and pick up the pieces and carry on.'

In Hollywood, Salma Hayek fought for her character in the film *The Hitman's Wife's Bodyguard* to be in her fifties and experiencing menopause, and it is set to be a theme in novels and TV shows. And in the Middle East, the incontinence company Tena campaigned to change the Arabic phrase for menopause from 'the age of despair' to 'the age of renewal'.

The knowledge I've gained from going through menopause and writing this book would have been helpful ten years ago. At the very least, I wouldn't have clenched my jaw in rage so much that it damaged my teeth. There would have been less sounding-off at strangers. Fewer tampons and pads. More sleep.

What I've learned has been complex and sometimes

contradictory, but the really important stuff can be summed up as follows:

- The focus on hot flushes is reductive — menopause is about far, FAR more than that.
- You shouldn't have to put up with having a worse life during the midlife transition. There are many things you can try.
- You are an individual, and your menopause experience won't be exactly the same as someone else's — so your treatment plan needs to be personalised, too.
- If people stand to make a lot of money from helping with your menopause symptoms, don't rush to give it to them. There are many low-cost options to try first. This is one area where you don't always get what you pay for.
- You might not always feel capable of doing the stuff you used to manage. Don't fight it. Don't feel bad. Just take the pressure off yourself if at all possible.
- More of anything is not necessarily better, whether it's dietary supplements, exercise or martinis.
- Talk to other midlife women, especially the ones who seem to be sailing through it — get them to reveal their secrets (whatever they are doing might not work for you, but it's KNOWLEDGE!).
- You don't have to be invisible unless you really want to, but you may need to embrace a vibrant new style.
- The secret to life is leafy green vegetables, but spinach

gets stuck in middle-aged teeth.

- Ageism is alive and well, the patriarchy is still in charge, more research is always needed, but CHANGE IS POSSIBLE.
- If you want a good life when you're elderly, you need to focus on living well in midlife.
- You don't have to cut your hair into a bob, let it go grey, cover your arms or midriff, or hide your tattoos ... but you can do all of those things if you want to.
- Midlife women have always had more wisdom and strength — now we also have more power.
- Like everything else in life, you'll have a better menopause experience if you prepare for it.
- Menopause isn't a time to dread or fear. Once you're through it, there are good things coming.

Writing a book about menopause while feeling very menopausal didn't always seem like the best idea. There were times when my confidence flagged and I felt entirely overwhelmed by the challenge. But I got there in the end, with the help of a lot of other women who generously and openly shared their stories and their knowledge. A big thank you is due to all of them.

I'm grateful to have had all those conversations. I feel enriched by them. The menopause revolution is about kōrero and mātauranga, whatever your culture, your age or your gender.

Not everybody who goes through menopause is a woman. Trans, intersex and non-binary people are on a journey that deserves a book of its own, and I'm not the writer who should tackle it. Disabled people, those with long-term health conditions, women battling serious illness — all change hormonally, too. While I've tried to reflect as much diversity as possible, there is more work to be done and lots more voices to be heard.

For all of us, no matter who we are, menopause is ephemeral, like any other stage of life. It's a coming-of-age, a time we're passing through, and we shouldn't have to do that silently.

I'm a writer, a horse rider, a vege gardener, a lover of food, a friend, a wife, a sister, a daughter. I'm not *only* menopausal and I don't want to be defined by that. But there's a revolution happening and I'm happy to be a part of it.

He waka eke noa — we're all in this together.

~

I'm giving the last word to journalist Carmen Parahi. I mention her earlier in the book as one of my dynamic midlife Kiwi women and when I emailed to check her age she came back with a long and fabulously inspiring message that she has kindly allowed me to use. It sums up a lot of what I'm thinking and feeling right now, and I might follow her example of drawing up a midlife to-do list:

I love being in my fifties. During my fiftieth year, I wrote a list of 50 things to do before I die. I turned 51 in August 2021 and I've already ticked one thing off the list.

I told some friends about my list. One of them, also in her fifties, remarked with surprise that I could still be ambitious at our age. My response was, 'Why wouldn't I?' Life ends when it ends. We shouldn't stop giving it a crack because we're in our fifties.

Both my parents, one over 70 and the other about to turn 70, still work in full-time manual jobs. They've got no intention of retiring. 'What for?' they reckon.

My list of 50 things to do is not a bucket list. I did that when I was in my teens. I wrote a list when I was 18 to achieve by 30 because I thought I'd be dead by then. Ah, youth. Thirty seemed so far away and really old. I ticked everything off the list, got to 30 and thought, 'Shite, now what?' Journalism. I've been in the adventure of journalism ever since.

So, in my fiftieth year I began to wonder. Could I live another 50 years? Maybe, probably not. But why not make it fun if I do? Actually, to be honest, my thought process went more like this: 'Fuck. I'm 50. I could live for another fucking 50 years! Fuck. I better sort my shit out.'

Don't Sweat it

My list is a mix of highly ambitious goals, like travelling to outer space, to less ambitious but equally important goals, such as being an expert doughnut maker. My kids and I collect sea glass, so I want to make jewellery from it for us and hopefully for my future, yet to arrive mokopuna, as a way to treasure those memories. Another is to create my own scent, so I can leave it for my children and mokopuna to remember me by. There are a few goals dedicated to service for others.

While I work fulltime and consider my 49 remaining goals, like millions of others worldwide, my body and mind are traversing te ruahinetanga or menopause. I'm fascinated by this natural process. Nature really is amazing, eh. I can feel the thickness at my waist, the hot flushes when they rush in. I laugh when my body burns up. I make a bit of a joke of it with my two teenage daughters to try to normalise it for them just as we do for mate wāhine, menstrual cycles. We celebrate these aspects of ourselves as something to be proud of, not to be talked or thought about in shame.

As a wāhine Māori, what does ruahinetanga mean for me now in my whānau roles and on the marae? I do not know. But to help understand what it could mean, it's important to keep learning, which is why I have a list of 50 things to do. I don't want to become rigid in my perspectives as I age. I prefer to remain flexible in my thinking by being open to new experiences, always in the pursuit of knowledge.

Women in their fifties are really terrific. We've got 50-odd damned years of experience, usually while working full-time, running a household and trying to make time for our personal lives. We've learned from those experiences. We know how to deal with a range of scenarios because we've probably already fucked it up, scored big or just scraped by. In our fifties it's a good time to provide leadership where we can because of our experiences. It gives us a been-there-done-that attitude, which is usually a mix of empathy and a I-don't-actually-give-a-fuck-about-your-reckons, haha.

Our fifties isn't a time to start feeling old. It really is an opportunity to reset, think and plan how you can add value to other peoples' lives and more importantly, what cracking adventures you could enjoy. Create a list of 50 ideas to do so you can stay agile in your body, mind and spirit. My list isn't complete yet, I purposefully left some spaces and I may amend some goals too. The point is it's something interesting to do with my time, it's purposeful and it's supposed to be fun.

After all, who doesn't love a great doughnut?

References

4. And then the menopause stole my personality (or at least borrowed it)

1   Circle In, 'Report: Menopause and the workplace', https://circlein.com/report-menopause-and-the-workplace.

2   R. Lewis & L. Newson, 'Menopause at work: A survey to look at the impact of menopausal and perimenopausal symptoms upon women in the workplace', My Menopause Doctor, available at www.menopausedoctor.co.uk/menopause/menopause-at-work-survey-results-1.

3   J. Horan, 'Menopause can be a battle, but the war is still about the patriarchy', *Ensemble*, (26 January 2021), https://www.ensemblemagazine.co.nz/articles/menopause-dr-jane-horan.

4   North American Menopause Society, 'Depression & Menopause', www.menopause.org/for-women/menopauseflashes/mental-health-at-menopause/depression-menopause.

5   F.N. Jacka, A. O'Neil, R. Opie, C. Itsiopoulos, S. Cotton, M. Mohebbi, D. Castle, . . . M.Berk, 'A randomised controlled trial of dietary improvement for adults with major depression (the "SMILES" trial)', *BMC Medicine*, vol. 15, no. 23 (2017), 23, DOI: 10.1186/s12916-017-0791-y.

6   T. Odai, M. Terauchi, A. Hirose, K. Kato, M. Akiyoshi & N. Miyasaka, 'Severity of hot flushes is inversely associated with dietary intake of vitamin B_6 and oily fish', *Climacteric*, vol. 22, no. 6 (2019), pp. 617–21, DOI: 10.1080/13697137.2019.1609440.

7   M.P. White, I. Alcock, J. Grellier, J. B.W. Wheeler, T. Hartig, S.L. Warber, A. Bone, . . . L.E. Fleming, 'Spending at least 120 minutes a week in nature is associated with good health and wellbeing', *Scientific Reports*, vol. 9 (2019), 7730, www.nature.com/articles/s41598-019-44097-3.

5. And then the menopause (hopefully) borrowed my libido

1   R.E. Nappi & M. Kokot-Kierepa, 'Vaginal health: Insights, Views & Attitudes (VIVA) — results from an international survey', *Climacteric*, vol. 15, no. 1 (February 2012), pp. 36–44, DOI: 10.3109/13697137.2011.647840.

2   Li FG, Maheux-Lacroix S, Deans R, et al. Effect of Fractional Carbon Dioxide Laser vs Sham Treatment on Symptom Severity in Women

With Postmenopausal Vaginal Symptoms: A Randomized Clinical Trial. JAMA. 2021;326(14):1381–1389. doi:10.1001/jama.2021.14892

3   S.R. Davis, R. Baber, N. Panay, J. Bitzer, S.C. Perez, R.M. Islam, A.M. Kaunitz, . . . M. E. Wierman, 'Global consensus position statement on the use of testosterone therapy for women', *Climacteric*, vol. 22, no. 5 (October 2019), pp. 429–34, DOI: 10.1080/13697137.2019.1637079. Available at www.imsociety.org/wp-content/uploads/2020/07/global-consensus-testosterone-english.pdf.

6. And then the menopause destroyed my superpower

1   A.A. Prather, D. Janicki-Deverts, M.H. Hall & S. Cohen, 'Behaviorally assessed sleep and susceptibility to the common cold', *Sleep*, vol. 38, no. 9 September 2015), pp. 1353–9, DOI: 10.5665/sleep.4968.

2   D.H. Solomon, K. Ruppert, L.A. Habel, J.S. Finkelstein, P. Lian, H. Joffe & H.M. Kravitz, 'Prescription medications for sleep disturbances among midlife women during 2 years of follow-up: A SWAN retrospective cohort study', *BMJ Open*, vol. 11, no. 5, e045074, DOI: 10.1136/bmjopen-2020-045074.

3   C. Drake, T. Roehrs, J. Shambroom & T. Roth, 'Caffeine effects on sleep taken 0, 3, or 6 hours before going to bed', *Journal of Clinical Sleep Medicine*, vol. 9, no. 11 (November 2013), pp. 1195–200, DOI: 10.5664/jcsm.3170.

7. It's also about progesterone

1   P. Schüssler, M. Kluge, A. Yassouridis, M. Dresler, K. Held, J. Zihl & A. Steiger, 'Progesterone reduces wakefulness in sleep EEG and has no effect on cognition in healthy postmenopausal women', *Psychoneuroendocrinology*, vol. 33, no. 8 (September 2008), pp. 1124–31, DOI: 10.1016/j.psyneuen.2008.05.013.

2   J.C. Prior, 'Progesterone for treatment of symptomatic menopausal women', *Climacteric*, vol. 21, no. 4 (August 2018), pp. 358–65, DOI: 10.1080/13697137.2018.1472567.

3   D. Grady, B. Ettinger, A.N.A. Tosteson, A. Pressman & J.L. Macer, 'Predictors of difficulty when discontinuing postmenopausal hormone therapy', *Obstetrics and Gynecology*, vol. 102, no. 6 December 2003), pp. 1233–39, DOI: 10.1016/j.obstetgynecol.2003.09.025.

4   Y. Fan, R. Tang, J.C. Prior & R. Chen, 'Paradigm shift in pathophysiology of vasomotor symptoms: Effects of estradiol withdrawal and progesterone therapy', *Drug Discovery Today: Disease Models*, vol. 32, part B (Winter 2020), pp. 59–69, DOI: 10.1016/j.ddmod.2020.11.004.

Don't Sweat it

5   J.C. Prior & C.L. Hitchcock, 'Progesterone for hot flush and night sweat treatment — effectiveness for severe vasomotor symptoms and lack of withdrawal rebound', *Gynecological Endocrinology*, vol. 28, suppl. 2 (October 2012), pp. 7–11, DOI: 10.3109/09513590.2012.705390.

6   A.H. Maclennan, J.L. Broadbent, S. Lester & V. Moore, 'Oral oestrogen and combined oestrogen/progestogen therapy versus placebo for hot flushes', *Cochrane Database of Systematic Reviews*, 2004, no. 4 (18 October 2004), CD002978, DOI: 10.1002/14651858.CD002978.pub2.

7   J.C. Prior, J.D. Nielsen, C.L. Hitchcock, L.A. Williams, Y.M. Vigna & C.B. Dean, 'Medroxyprogesterone and conjugated oestrogen are equivalent for hot flushes: A 1-year randomized double-blind trial following premenopausal ovariectomy', *Clinical Science (London)*, vol. 112, no. 10 (May 2007), pp. 517–25, DOI: 10.1042/cs20060266.

8   J.C. Prior, 'Women's reproductive system as balanced estradiol and progesterone actions—a revolutionary, paradigm-shifting concept in women's health', *Drug Discovery Today: Disease Models*, vol. 32, part B (Winter 2020), pp. 31–40, DOI: 10.1016/j.ddmod.2020.11.005.

8. Why is it all so hard? (A short history of HRT)

1   J.E. Rossouw, G.L. Anderson, R.L. Prentice, A.Z. LaCroix, C. Kooperberg, M.L. Stefanick, R.D Jackson ... Writing Group for the Women's Health Initiative Investigators, 'Risks and benefits of estrogen plus progestin in healthy postmenopausal women: Principal results from the Women's Health Initiative randomized controlled trial. *JAMA*, vol. 288, no. 3 (17 July 2002), pp. 321–33, DOI: 10.1001/jama.288.3.321.

2   L.R. Newson & R. Langer, 'Trying to right 20 years of misinformation and hysteria about HRT — Professor Rob Lander and Dr Louise Newson', My Menopause Doctor, www.menopausedoctor.co.uk/menopause/097-trying-to-right-20-years-of-misinformation-and-hysteria-about-hrt-professor-rob-langer-and-dr-louise-newson.

3   Collaborative Group on Hormonal Factors in Breast Cancer, 'Type and timing of menopausal hormone therapy and breast cancer risk: Individual participant meta-analysis of the worldwide epidemiological evidence', *Lancet*, vol. 394, no. 10204 (28 September 2019), pp. 1159–68, DOI: 10.1016/S0140-6736(19)31709-X.

4   J. Rymer, K. Brian & L. Regan, 'HRT and breast cancer risk', *BMJ*, vol. 367 (11 October 2019), l5928, DOI: 10.1136/bmj.l5928.

5   Australasian Menopause Society, 'Risks and benefits of MHT' (Information sheet) (2021), available at www.menopause.org.au/hp/information-sheets/risks-and-benefits-of-mht-hrt.

6   S.J. Lowry, K. Kapphahn, R. Chlebowski & C.I. Li, 'Alcohol use and

breast cancer survival among participants in the Women's Health Initiative', *Cancer Epidemiology Biomarkers & Prevention*, vol. 25, no. 8 (August 2016), pp. 1268–73, DOI: 10.1158/1055-9965.EPI-16-0151.

7   World Cancer Research Fund & American Institute for Cancer Research, 'Diet, nutrition, physical activity and breast cancer', (2017, revised 2018), www.wcrf.org/wp-content/uploads/2021/02/Breast-cancer-report.pdf.

10. Food: friend or foe?

1   T. Yang, J. Doherty, B. Zhao, A.J. Kinchia, J.M. Clark & L. He, 'Effectiveness of commercial and homemade washing agents in removing pesticide residues on and in apples', *Journal of Agricultural and Food Chemistry*, vol. 65, no. 4 (2017), pp. 9744–52, DOI: 10.1021/acs.jafc.7b03118.

2   A.N. Gearhardt, S. Yokum, P.T. Orr, E. Stice, W.R. Corbin & K.D. Brownell, 'Neural correlates of food addiction', *Archives of General Psychiatry*, vol. 68, no. 8 (August 2011), pp. 808–16, DOI: 10.1001/archgenpsychiatry.2011.32.

3   Kenny & Johnson 'Addiction: Junk-food junkies', *Nature*, vol. 464, no. 652 (2010), https://doi.org/10.1038/464652c.

4   S. Mackay, C. Ni Mhurchu, B. Swinburn, H. Eyles, L. Young & T. Gontijo de Castro, 'State of the food supply New Zealand 2019' (online resource), Auckland, The University of Auckland, https://doi.org/10.17608/k6.auckland.9636710.v1.

5   M.E.J. Lean, W.S. Leslie, A.C. Barnes, N. Brosnahan, G. Thom, Louise McCombie, C. Peters, . . . R. Taylor, 'Primary care-led weight management for remission of type 2 diabetes (DiRECT): An open-label, cluster-randomised trial', *Lancet*, vol. 391, no. 10120 (10 February 2018), pp. 541–51, DOI: 10.1016/S0140-6736(17)33102-1.

6   E. Fothergill, J. Guo, L. Howard, J.C. Kerns, N.D. Knuth, R. Brytcha, K.Y. Chen, . . . K.D. Hall, 'Persistent metabolic adaptation 6 years after "The Biggest Loser" competition', *Obesity (Silver Spring)*, vol. 24, no. 8 (August 2016), pp. 1612–19, DOI: 10.1002/oby.21538.

7   S. Berry, A. Valdes, R. Davies, L. Delahunty, D. Drew, A.T. Chan, N. Segata, . . . T. Spector, 'Predicting personal metabolic responses to food using multi-omics machine learning in over 1000 twins and singletons from the UK and US: The PREDICT I Study (OR31-01-19)', *Current Developments in Nutrition*, vol. 3, suppl. 1 (June 2019), nzz037.OR31-01-19, DOI: 10.1093/cdn/nzz037.OR31-01-19,

8   T. Odai, M. Terauchi, A. Hirose, K. Kato, M. Akiyoshi & N. Miyasaka, 'Severity of hot flushes is inversely associated with dietary intake of

vitamin B$_6$ and oily fish', *Climacteric*, vol. 22, no. 6 (December 2019), pp. 617–21, DOI: 10.1080/13697137.2019.1609440.

9   N.D. Barnard, H. Kahleova, D.N. Holtz, F. Del Aguila, M. Neola, L.M. Crosby & R. Holubkov, 'The Women's Study for the Alleviation of Vasomotor Symptoms (WAVS): A randomized, controlled trial of a plant-based diet and whole soybeans for postmenopausal women', *Menopause*, (12 July 2021) (Epub ahead of print), DOI: 10.1097/GME.0000000000001812.

11. Out of our way, we're coming through

1   Forbes, 'Forbes presents 50 over 50 [know your value]', /www.forbes.com/50over50.

12. I want to feel like a natural woman

1   Australasian Menopause Society, 'Bioidentical custom compounded hormone therapy' (Information sheet), available at www.menopause.org.au/hp/information-sheets/bioidentical-hormones-for-menopausal-symptoms.

2   P.A. Komesaroff, C.V. Black, V. Cable & K. Sudhir, 'Effects of wild yam extract on menopausal symptoms, lipids and sex hormones in healthy menopausal women', *Climacteric*, vol. 4, no. 2 (June 2001), pp. 144–50, PMID: 11428178.

3   M.J. Leach & V. Moore, 'Black cohosh (*Cimicifuga* spp.) for menopausal symptoms', *Cochrane Library of Systematic Reviews*, (2012), CD007244, www.cochranelibrary.com/cdsr/doi/10.1002/14651858.CD007244.pub2/full.

4   M. Mehrpooya, S. Rabiee, A. Larki-Harchegani, A.-M. Fallahian, A. Moradi, S. Ataei & M.T. Javad, 'A comparative study on the effect of "black cohosh" and "evening primrose oil" on menopausal hot flashes', *Journal of Education and Health Promotion*, vol. 7 (1 March 2018), p. 36, DOI: 10.4103/jehp.jehp_81_17.

5   Royal New Zealand College of General Practioners, www.rnzcgp.org.nz/RNZCGP/News/College_news/2021/College_of_GPs_releases_latest_Workforce_Survey_data.aspx

6   North American Menopause Society. 'Nonhormonal management of menopause-associated vasomotor symptoms: 2015 position statement of The North American Menopause Society', *Menopause*, vol. 22, no. 11 (2015), pp. 1155–74, DOI: 10.1097/GME.0000000000000546. Available at www.menopause.org/docs/default-source/professional/2015-nonhormonal-therapy-position-statement.pdf.

7   North American Menopause Society, 'More women using cannabis for menopause symptoms' [press release], 22 September 2021,

www.menopause.org/docs/default-source/press-release/cannabis-use-for-menopause-symptoms.pdf.

8   A.L. Lopresti, S.J. Smith, H. Malvi & R. Kodgule, 'An investigation into the stress-relieving and pharmacological actions of an ashwagandha (*Withania somnifera*) extract: A randomized, double-blind, placebo-controlled study', *Medicine*, vol. 98, no. 37 (September 2019), e17186, DOI: 10.1097/MD.0000000000017186.

13. Hearts & Minds & Bones

1   M.J. Stampfer, G.A. Colditz, W.C. Willett, J.E. Manson, B. Rosner, F.E. Speizer & C.H. Hennekens, 'Postmenopausal estrogen therapy and cardiovascular disease. Ten-year follow-up from the Nurses' Health Study', *New England Journal of Medicine*, vol. 325, no. 11 (12 September 1991), pp. 756–62, DOI: 10.1056/NEJM199109123251102.

2   M. Venetkoski, H. Savolainen-Peltonen, P. Rahkola-Soisalo, F. Hoti, P. Vattulainen, M. Gissler, O. Ylikorkala & T.S. Mikkola, 'Increased cardiac and stroke death risk in the first year after discontinuation of postmenopausal hormone therapy', *Menopause*, vol. 25, no. 4 (April 2018), pp. 375–9, DOI: 10.1097/GME.0000000000001023.

3   L. Mosconi, V. Berti, J. Dyke, E. Schelbaum, S. Jett, L. Loughlin, G. Jang, . . . R. Diaz Brinton, 'Menopause impacts human brain structure, connectivity, energy metabolism, and amyloid-beta deposition', *Scientific Reports*, vol. 11 (2021), 10867, DOI: 10.1038/s41598-021-90084-y.

4   Nuffield Health, 'One in four with menopause symptoms concerned about ability to cope with life', Nuffield Health (14 September 2017), https://www.nuffieldhealth.com/article/one-in-four-with-menopause-symptoms-concerned-about-ability-to-cope-with-life.

5   Y.J. Kim, M. Soto, G.L Branigan, K. Rodgers & R. Diaz Brinton, 'Association between menopausal hormone therapy and risk of neurodegenerative diseases: Implications for precision hormone therapy', *Alzheimer's & Dementia (New York)*, vol. 7, no. 1 ((2021), e12174, DOI: 10.1002/trc2.12174.

6   G. Livingston, J. Huntley, A. Sommerlad, D. Ames, C. Ballard, S. Banerjee, C. Brayne, . . . N. Mukadam, 'Dementia prevention, intervention, and care: 2020 report of the *Lancet* Commission', *Lancet*, vol. 396, no. 10248 (8 August 2020), pp. 413–46, DOI: 10.1016/S0140-6736(20)30367-6.

7   M.J. Bolland, W. Leung, V. Tai, S. Bastin, G.D. Gamble, A. Grey & I.R. Reid, 'Calcium intake and risk of fracture: Systematic review', *BMJ*, vol. 351 (2015), h4580, DOI: 10.1136/bmj.h4580.

8   J. Wise, 'Vitamin D supplementation to prevent osteoporosis is not warranted, study concludes', *BMJ*, vol. 347 (2013), f6156, DOI: 10.1136/bmj.f6156.

9   S.E. Reuter, H.B. Schultz, M.B. Ward, C.L. Grant, G.M. Paech, S. Banks & A.M. Evans, 'The effect of high-dose, short-term caffeine intake on the renal clearance of calcium, sodium and creatinine in healthy adults', *British Journal of Clinical Pharmacology*, (14 April 2021) (Epub ahead of print), DOI: 10.1111/bcp.14856.

10 Ministry of Health Manatū Hauora, 'Vitamin D', www.health.govt.nz/your-health/healthy-living/food-activity-and-sleep/healthy-eating/vitamin-d.

11 S.L. Watson, B.K. Weeks, L.J. Weis, A.T. Harding, S.A. Horan & B.R. Beck, 'High-intensity resistance and impact training improves bone mineral density and physical function in postmenopausal women with osteopenia and osteoporosis: The LIFTMOR randomized controlled trial', *Journal of Bone and Mineral Research*, vol. 33, no. 2 (February 2018), pp. 211–20, DOI: 10.1002/jbmr.3284. Erratum in: *Journal of Bone and Mineral Research*, vol. 34, no. 3 (March 2019), p. 572.

14. Why OK Boomer is not OK

1   Human Rights Commission Te Kāhui Tiki Tangata in partnership with the Office for Senior Citizens Te Tari Kaumātua & OCG Consulting, 'Ageing workforce in the New Zealand Crown Entity sector: Survey report 2014', www.hrc.co.nz/files/4414/2357/1973/NZ-Crown-Entity-Sector-Ageing-Workforce-White-Paper-November-2014.doc.

16. Exercise to energise, not exhaust

1   A.V. Patel, M.L. Maliniak, E. Rees-Punia, C.E. Matthews & S.M. Gapstur, 'Prolonged leisure time spent sitting in relation to cause-specific mortality in a large US cohort', *American Journal of Epidemiology*, vol. 187, no. 10 (October 2018), pp. 2151–8, DOI: 10.1093/aje/kwy125.

2   H, Hörder, L. Johansson, X.-X. Guo, G. Grimby, S. Kern, S. Östling & I. Skooog, 'Midlife cardiovascular fitness and dementia: A 44-year longitudinal population study in women', *Neurology*, vol. 90, no. 15 (April 2018), e1298–e1305, DOI: 10.1212/WNL.0000000000005290.

3   K.J. Gries, U. Raue, R.K. Perkins, K.M. Lavin, B.S. Overstreet, L.J. D'Acquisto, B. Graham, . . . S. Trappe, 'Cardiovascular and skeletal muscle health with lifelong exercise', *Journal of Applied Physiology*, vol 25, no. 1 (1 November 2018), pp. 1636–45, DOI: 10.1152/japplphysiol.00174.2018.

4   C. Hartley, J.P. Folland, R. Kerslake & K. Brooke-Wavell, 'High-impact exercise increased femoral neck bone density with no adverse effects on imaging markers of knee osteoarthritis in postmenopausal women', *Journal of Bone and Mineral Research*, vol. 35, no. 1 (January 2020), pp. 53–63, DOI: 10.1002/jbmr.3867.

17. Some thoughts on men

1   Statistics New Zealand Tatauranga Aotearoa, 'Marriages, civil unions, and divorces: Year ended December 2019', (May 2020), www.stats.govt. nz/information-releases/marriages-civil-unions-and-divorces-year-ended-december-2019.

18. Inflammation, telomeres and the science of ageing well

1   M. Tamez, A. Monge, R. López-Ridaura, G. Fagherazzi, S. Rinaldi, E. Ortiz-Panozo, E. Yunes, . . . M. Lajous, 'Soda intake is directly associated with serum C-reactive protein concentration in Mexican women', *Journal of Nutrition*, vol. 148, no. 1 (January 2018), pp. 117–124, DOI: 10.1093/jn/nxx021.

2   E.S. Epel, E.H. Blackburn, J. Lin, F.S. Dhabhar, N.E. Adler, J.D. Morrow & R.M. Cawthon, 'Accelerated telomere shortening in response to life stress', *Proceedings of the National Academy of Science of the United States of America*, vol. 101, no. 49 (7 December 2004), pp. 17312–15, DOI: 10.1073/pnas.0407162101.

3   H. Lavretsky, P. Siddarth, N. Nazarian, N. St. Cyr, D.S. Khalsa, J. Lin, E. Blackburn, . . . M.R. Irwin. 'A pilot study of yogic meditation for family dementia caregivers with depressive symptoms: Effects on mental health, cognition, and telomerase activity', *International Journal of Geriatric Psychiatry*, vol. 28, no. 1 (January 2013), pp. 57–65, DOI: 10.1002/gps.3790.

4   D.S.T. Cheung, W. Deng, S.-W. Tsao, R.T.H. Ho, C.L.W. Chan, D.Y.T. Fong, P.H. Chau, . . . A.F.Y. Tiwari. 'Effect of a qigong intervention on telomerase activity and mental health in Chinese women survivors of intimate partner violence: A randomized clinical trial', *JAMA Network Open*, vol. 2, no. 1 (2019), e186967, DOI: 10.1001/jamanetworkopen.2018.6967.

19. And so to sum up

1   E. Hinchliffe, 'Menopause is a $600 billion opportunity, report finds', *Fortune*, (27 October 2020), https://fortune.com/2020/10/26/menopause-startups-female-founders-fund-report.

Further reading

Books
Sam Baker, *The Shift: How I (lost and) found myself after 40 — and you can too*, Coronet, 2021.

Joanna Blythman, *Swallow This: Serving up the food industry's darkest secrets*, Fourth Estate, 2015.

Laura Briden, *Hormone Repair Manual: Every woman's guide to healthy hormones after 40*, Greenpeak Publishing, 2021.

Louise Foxcroft, *Hot Flushes, Cold Science: A history of the modern menopause*, Granta UK, 2010.

Jen Gunter, *The Menopause Manifesto: Own your health with facts and feminism*, Citadel Press, 2021.

Ginni Mansberg, *The M Word: How to thrive in menopause*, Murdoch Books, 2020.

Articles
Dr Jane Horan, 'Menopause can be a battle, but the war is still about the patriarchy', *Ensemble*, 26 January 2021, www.ensemblemagazine.co.nz/articles/menopause-dr-jane-horan

Suzanne Moore, 'There won't be blood: Suzanne Moore on the menopause', *New Statesman*, 17 August 2015, www.newstatesman.com/lifestyle/2015/08/there-wont-be-blood-suzanne-moore-menopause

Useful websites
Australasian Menopause Society
www.menopause.org.au/
NZ doctors who are members:
www.menopause.org.au/health-info/find-an-ams-doctor/new-zealand

Best Practice Advocacy Centre New Zealand (bpac^{NZ})
bpac.org.nz

CeMCOR (the Centre for Menstrual Cycle and Ovulation Research)
www.cemcor.ca

Cochrane Library
www.cochranelibrary.com

International Menopause Society
www.imsociety.org

Menopause Over Martinis

www.menopauseovermartinis.org
Menopause Support UK
  menopausesupport.co.uk
Mementia
  www.mentemia.com
My Menopause Doctor
  www.menopausedoctor.co.uk
North American Menopause Society
  www.menopause.org

Index